THE ROLE OF THE CLINICAL CARDIAC ELECTROPHYSIOLOGIST IN THE MANAGEMENT OF CONGESTIVE HEART FAILURE

Edited by **John Kassotis**

The Role of the Clinical Cardiac Electrophysiologist in the Management of Congestive Heart Failure
http://dx.doi.org/10.5772/63292
Edited by John Kassotis

Contributors

Gabriel Cismaru, Lucian Muresan, Mihai Puiu, Radu Rosu, Gabriel Gusetu, Dana Pop, Dumitru Zdrenghea, Daryl Irving Smith, Albert Duah, Takashi Murashita, Massimo Grimaldi, Antonio Di Monaco, Federico Quadrini, Nicola Vitulano, Guillermo Mora, Miguel Ángel García García, Adina Stanciu, Adina Zamfir-Chiru-Anton, Marcel Stanciu, Dan-Cristian Gheorghe, Jeffrey Stephen Borer, Oleg Yurevich

Published by InTech
Janeza Trdine 9, 51000 Rijeka, Croatia

Publishing Process Manager Ana Simcic
Technical Editor SPi Global
Cover InTech Design team

First published February, 2017
Printed in Croatia
Legal deposit, Croatia: National and University Library in Zagreb

Additional hard copies can be obtained from orders@intechopen.com

The Role of the Clinical Cardiac Electrophysiologist in the Management of Congestive Heart Failure, Edited by John Kassotis
p. cm.
Print ISBN 978-953-51-2947-9
Online ISBN 978-953-51-2948-6

For EU product safety concerns:
IN TECH d.o.o., Prolaz Marije Krucifikse Kozulić 3, 51000 Rijeka, Croatia, info@intechopen.com or visit our website at intechopen.com.

Meet the editor

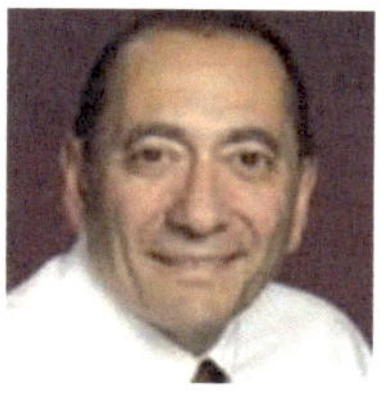

Dr. John Kassotis received his doctorate in chemical engineering from the Columbia University, School of Engineering and Applied Sciences, in 1985 and earned his MD degree from the Columbia College of Physicians and Surgeons in 1990. After completing his residency, cardiovascular fellowship, and electrophysiology fellowship at the Presbyterian Hospital, Dr. Kassotis began the Arrhythmia Service at New York Methodist Hospital (clinical affiliate of the NY Presbyterian Hospital Network) where he served as the director. In 2005, Dr. Kassotis was appointed the director of the Clinical Cardiac Electrophysiology Section and Fellowship Programs at SUNY Downstate Medical Center. He has authored or coauthored over 70 peer-reviewed articles, book chapters, and patents. He is the recipient of multiple teaching awards and serves as associate editor of the journal Cardiology.

Contents

Preface

The impetus to write a textbook exploring the role of the clinical cardiac electrophysiologist, in the management of systolic heart failure, arose from a genuine interest in more intimately managing my patients with congestive heart failure. It became apparent that there was a lack of a streamline exchange of information, between the heart failure specialists and the electrophysiology service.

This inspired me to become boarded not only in clinical cardiac electrophysiology but also in advanced heart failure and cardiac transplantation. This furthered my appreciation of how important it has become for these two disciplines to work hand in hand. This inspired me to create a textbook, which explored the role of the clinical cardiac electrophysiologists in the management of systolic heart failure.

Electrophysiology has experienced a remarkable evolution. From the early days of using an intravascular catheter to recording a His Bundle, better identifying patients in need of permanent pacing to the use of a similarly designed intravascular catheter to ablate the focus of a plethora of arrhythmias. This enabled us to better identify, understand, and more definitively treat the wide variety of arrhythmia we encounter in clinical medicine. Over the past decade with refinements in imaging technologies, we have expanded our armamentarium to more complex rhythm disturbances, effectively treating atrial fibrillation and complex ventricular tachycardia. These advances have resulted not only in mortality benefits but also in improved quality of life.

Equally remarkable is the evolution of the cardiac devices. From the first-generation pacemaker and the first implantable cardioverter defibrillator (ICD), we now have devices that integrate both technologies. From a cumbersome extracorporeal device, to a simple pacing and ICD system, we have now integrated these two technologies and incorporating a strategically placed coronary sinus lead to resynchronize the right and left ventricles in patients with systolic heart failure and a left bundle branch block. This has had a major impact on the morbidity and mortality of an ever-expanding population.

Although a great deal remains to be learned, in particular what will be the role of the electrophysiologist in the management of the arrhythmic issues faced by patients following the insertion of a left ventricular assist device (LVAD). With a reduction in available donor hearts and an expanded role of the (LVAD) destination therapy will have an ever-expanding role in managing these patients. This will undoubtedly expand the critical role of the electrophysiologists in the management of these complex patients.

The impetus of this textbook is to reinforce the electrophysiologists and their colleagues in advanced heart failure the synergistic roles they introduce in the management of these very complex patients. It also serves as a stepping stone to what I truly believe will be a growing body of literature.

The textbook is organized in four sections:

Section 1 explores newer pharmacology and novel therapeutic techniques in the treatment of systolic heart failure. Section 2 focuses on the role of implantable devices in the management of systolic heart failure including the impact of cardiac resynchronization therapy (CRT), addressing who is most likely to respond and how we can optimize this response. Section 3 discusses the role of transcatheter ablative therapy in the management of atrial fibrillation and other arrhythmias in patients with heart failure. The final section looks at the impact of thyroid disease in congestive heart failure.

I want to extend a heartfelt thank you to the collection of international authors who contributed to this textbook, without whom this textbook would not have been possible. It is my hope that the textbook will meet its stated objective and will serve as the fodder for physicians at all levels of training to appreciate the intimate role of the these two important disciplines of cardiovascular medicine.

I would like to extend a thank you to Carolyn my partner in crime who had to endure endless hours without me while I was preparing this book. I also want to thank my twin daughters Alexis and Denae who are busy with Medical and Law schools, respectively, and had to endure my lateness to many social engagements. Without everyone's patience, this book would not have been possible.

Dr. John Kassotis

Director of Clinical Cardiac Electrophysiology Section and Fellowship Program

SUNY Downstate Medical Center

New York, USA

Section 1

Pharmacology and Novel Therapeutic Techniques for Treatment of Systolic Heart Failure

Chapter 1

Role of New Therapies in Reducing Mortality and Major Morbidity in Patients with Systolic Heart Failure

Oleg Yurevich and Jeffrey S. Borer

Additional information is available at the end of the chapter

http://dx.doi.org/10.5772/66284

Abstract

Though heart failure therapies, particularly for systolic heart failure, have developed rapidly and markedly during the past four decades, a need for additional relief persists and is progressively being met. Two new drugs have been approved for marketing in the United States within the past two years, and two other glucose lowering therapies for diabetes appear to have efficacy for heart failure as well. In addition, device therapy for heart failure has progressed markedly during the past 5 years, particularly in refinements of the indications and applications of devices to minimize symptoms and hospitalizations and to maximize survival. This chapter will outline these recent developments.

Keywords: cardiovascular pharmacology, cardiovascular devices, angiotensin receptor blocker neprilysin inhibitor (ARNI), heart rate slowing, glucagon-like peptide receptor agonist

1. Introduction

Heart failure affects almost 6 million Americans [1], of whom 1 million are hospitalized for heart failure annually [2]. According to latest available data published in June 2016 in the National Vital Statistics Report, in 2014 cardiovascular diseases were the leading causes of death in the United States, responsible for 803,227 deaths of which 68,626 (8.5%) were related to heart failure [3]. Recent therapeutic advances suggest the potential for important amelioration of these outcomes when the new therapies are added to conventional modalities. In this chapter we will review the recent data supporting the incorporation of these new therapies into clinical practice.

2. Ivabradine

In April 2015, FDA approved ivabradine for reduction of heart failure hospitalizations for patients with heart failure with reduced ejection fraction (HFrEF) [4].

Ivabradine selectively blocks sinoatrial nodal cell hyperpolarization-activated cyclic nucleotide-gated (HCN) channels and, consequently, blocks the resulting transmembrane current (I_f) by entering and binding to a site in the channel pore from the intracellular side [5, 6]. In the United States, it is currently indicated for reduction in heart failure hospitalizations in patients with symptomatic chronic heart failure with ejection fraction ≤35% who are in sinus rhythm, with heart rate ≥70 beats per minute who already are being treated with maximally tolerated β-blockade [7] (as well as other conventional drugs for HFrEF). The drug now is recommended in the updated AHA-ACC guidelines for treatment of patients with HFrEF (class IIa recommendation, level of evidence B-R) [8]. In several other countries, the drug also is indicated for reduction in mortality or heart failure hospitalizations in patients with HFrEF, and also to prevent angina pectoris in symptomatic patients with chronic stable coronary artery disease irrespective of heart failure.

Ivabradine is unique in that it targets the HCN channel subtype found predominantly in sinoatrial nodal cells [9] and, thus, has little effect elsewhere in the heart or in other tissues (though drug action on HCN channels in the retina, similar to those in the sinoatrial node, is believed to underlie the side effect of visual phosphenes [flashing scotomata] reported in 3% of patients in the Systolic Heart Failure Treatment With the I_f Inhibitor Ivabradine Trial [SHIFT]). This locus of activity differs from that of β-blockers, which also slow heart rate but act wherever β-receptors are present (e.g., in the ventricles, causing negative inotropy, in the bronchi, causing bronchoconstriction, etc.) and from calcium channel blockers, the action of which, in the heart and smooth muscle, can cause negative inotropy, hypotension, and constipation. Ivabradine is a selective and specific inhibitor of the myocardial I_f, a current involved in modulating the cardiac pacemaker current [10]. At therapeutic concentrations, both in animals and humans, ivabradine does not affect any other cardiac channel or current (including those involving Na^+, K^+, or Ca^{2+}) [6].

To be active, ivabradine needs to penetrate the HCN channels; this requires appropriate orientation of the channel components, which occurs when the channel is hyperpolarized to [-40 mV]. Thus, the relevant channels are hyperpolarization-activated. As heart rate increases, the time during which the channels are hyperpolarized, and thus open to ivabradine, increases. Consequently, ivabradine-mediated heart rate reduction is "use dependent," i.e., it is more pronounced as heart rate increases [9].

Dosage: The evidence-based and recommended maximal dose of ivabradine is 7.5 mg twice daily [11]; the recommended starting dose of 5 mg twice daily.

Clinical evidence: Evidence supporting the utility of ivabradine for HFrEF primarily derives from SHIFT. The study was an event-driven, multinational, randomized, double-blinded, parallel-group trial in patients in sinus rhythm with heart rate ≥70 beats/min with moderate-to-severe heart failure and left ventricular ejection fraction ≤35% [11].

The study involved 6505 patients (53 of the original 6558 patients were censored for a major protocol violation) from 677 centers in 37 countries. Participants were randomized to ivabradine titrated to a maximum of 7.5 mg twice daily or to matched placebo and were followed for a median of 22.9 months and a maximum of 42 months [11, 13].

Study subjects were at least 18 years old (male and female) with symptomatically stable heart failure (and drug therapy) for at least 4 weeks and a hospitalization for worsening heart failure within the previous 12 months [11].

Treatment with ivabradine was associated with a placebo-subtracted average reduction in heart rate of 10.9 bpm at 1 month after randomization and 9.1 bpm at 1 year. The SHIFT primary composite endpoint (cardiovascular death or first hospitalization for worsening heart failure) was reduced by 18% (hazard ratio, 0.82 [95% CI, 0.75–0.90], $p < 0.0001$), driven primarily by reduction in hospitalizations for worsening heart failure (26% reduction, hazard ration, 0.74 [95% CI, 0.66–0.83], $p < 0.0001$). Death from heart failure fell to 26% (hazard ratio, 0.74 [95% CI, 0.58–0.94], $p = 0.014$).

From 1 year onward, at least 70% of patients were at the target dose of ivabradine (7.5 mg twice daily). By contrast, only 49% of the 6505 patients enrolled in the trial were able to reach at least 50% of evidence-based target β-blocker dose at baseline (90% were receiving at least some dose of beta blocker) because of contraindications or poor tolerability [11].

Cardiovascular and all-cause deaths were not significantly reduced by ivabradine [11], though, numerically, a 9% reduction in cardiovascular death was observed in the ivabradine group. (However, in Europe, the European Medicines Agency ordered a reanalysis of the data with entry at heart rate ≥75 bpm. This analysis revealed significant reduction in mortality as well as in hospitalizations. As a result, approval in Europe is for patients with symptomatic heart failure and LVEF ≤35% in sinus rhythm with heart rate ≥75 bpm.)

Sudden cardiac death was not affected by ivabradine, perhaps because of the effect of the background β-blocker treatment, which, unlike ivabradine, has intrinsic electrophysiological effects and is known to affect sudden cardiac death [11].

Postulated mechanisms of benefit from ivabradine-mediated heart rate reduction include decreased myocyte ischemia, improving the balance between myocardial oxygen (and energy) supply and demand; this effect is attributable not only to reduction in demand but also to increased supply caused by lengthening duration of diastole during which coronary flow occurs, and lack of negative lusitropy (relaxation, an active process that is inhibited by ischemia and also by beta blockade) reducing impedance to coronary flow relative to beta blockade [12]; other data suggest that use of the drug also increases endothelial cell proliferation, endothelial nitric oxide synthase (eNOS) activity, and increased collateral function [13].

The most prominent adverse effects of ivabradine are excessive bradycardia [14–16], atrial fibrillation [14, 15], and phosphenes (visual brightness in one portion of the visual field) [15, 16], and a small but significant increase in systolic blood pressure (the clinical importance of which is not clear) [15]. In SHIFT, the drug was not studied in patients with acute decompensated heart failure and thus is not indicated for such patients, through recent data [17, 18] suggest that beginning the drug early during a hospitalization for acute decompensated heart failure is acceptably safe and is effective in lowering heart rate. The drug also is contraindicated in patients with blood pressure less than 90/50 mmHg, and in the presence of sick sinus syndrome, sinoatrial block, or third degree AV block, unless a functioning demand pacemaker is present, and in patients with severe hepatic impairment or concomitant use of strong cytochrome P450 3A4 (CYP3A4) inhibitors or enhancers (ivabradine is metabolized in the liver by the P450 CYP 3A4 system). Because the target heart rate (supported by the SHIFT data [11]) is 50–60 bpm, the drug should not be given if the pretherapy heart rate already is ≤60 bpm; also, ivabradine is contraindicated (because it would have no effect) in patients who are pacemaker dependent (heart rate maintained exclusively by the pacemaker). Animal studies indicate the potential for fetal cardiac malformations if given during pregnancy [15]; therefore, its use is contraindicated during pregnancy and, if used in nonpregnant women of child-bearing age, effective contraception should be assured. At doses up to 10 mg BID, ivabradine prolongs the uncorrected QT interval; however, when appropriately corrected for heart rate, this increase does not exceed 2 ms, precluding direct proarrhythmic potential [16].

3. Sacubitril-valsartan

In July 2015, a few months after approval of ivabradine, FDA approved sacubitril-valsartan, also for treatment of patients with HFrEF [19].

Sacubitril-valsartan is a combination of an already approved angiotensin receptor blocker (valsartan) and a neprilysin inhibitor (such combination drugs are now known as ARNIs).

Neprilysin is a neutral endopeptidase and plays an important role in pathogenesis of heart failure and hypertension by catalyzing the degradation of endogenous vasoactive peptides, such as atrial natriuretic peptide (ANP), brain natriuretic peptide (BNP), C-type natriuretic peptide (CNP), endothelin-1 (ET-1), angiotensin II, and bradykinin [20]. Inhibition of neprilysin raises blood concentrations of these vasoactive peptides, some of which have potentially beneficial hemodynamic effects in patients with heart failure [20].

Inhibition of this neutral endopeptidase promotes sodium and water excretion by inhibiting sodium reabsorption in the proximal and distal nephron [21], and can cause reduction in systemic vascular resistance, pulmonary artery pressure, and pulmonary capillary wedge pressure. Blockage of neprilysin is associated with arterial stiffness reduction, enhanced endothelial function, and cardiac antihypertrophic and antifibrotic effects [13, 21]. Sacubitril-valsartan also has inhibitory actions on the renin-angiotensin-aldosterone system and sympathetic nervous system [13, 21].

FDA has approved marketing of the new ARNI for reduction in mortality and heart failure hospitalizations in patients with chronic heart failure (NYHA Class II–IV) and at least moderately subnormal ejection fraction (<40%) and the AHA-ACC Updated Heart Failure Guideline recommend its use for this indication [8, 22]. In patients with chronic symptomatic HFrEF NYHA class II or III who tolerate an ACE inhibitor or ARB, replacement by an ARNI

http://dx.doi.org/10.5772/66284

is guideline-recommended to further reduce morbidity and mortality (strength of recommendation I and level of evidence B-R) [8].

Dosage: The initial dose of 24/26 mg twice daily is recommended for patients not currently taking an ACE inhibitor or an angiotensin II receptor blocker (ARB) and for patients previously taking low doses of these agents. The dose can be doubled every 2–4 weeks, as tolerated, to reach the target maintenance dose of 97/103 mg twice daily [22].

Clinical evidence: The evidence supporting the efficacy of this ARNI was shown in the Prospective Comparison of ARNI With ACEi to Determine Impact on Global Mortality and Morbidity in Heart Failure (PARADIGM-HF) trial [23].

The study included 8442 randomized patients with chronic heart failure (NYHA Class II–IV) and ejection fraction ≤40%. Patients received either a combination of valsartan and sacubitril (200 mg [97/103 mg] twice daily) or the ACE inhibitor enalapril (10 mg twice daily) in addition to other guidelines-recommended therapy. The trial was stopped early due to highly significant benefit of sacubitril-valsartan without excessive adversity.

The composite endpoint (cardiovascular death and heart failure hospitalizations) was reduced by 20%, as were both components of this endpoint (CV death reduction: hazard ratio, 0.80 [95% CI, 0.71–0.89] $p < 0.001$, heart failure hospitalizations reduction: hazard ratio, 0.79 [95% CI, 0.71–0.89] $p < 0.001$). Death from any cause also was reduced by sacubitril-valsartan by 16% ($p < 0.001$).

During PARADIGM-HF most adverse events were more frequent on the already approved enalapril than on the ARNI combination drug. Of those of greatest concern (hypotension, renal insufficiency, angioedema, and hyperkalemia) only hypotension was significantly more frequent with sacubitril-valsartan, while angioedema, though more frequent with the combination (and known to be a potential consequence of neprilysin inhibition), occurred relatively infrequently [8, 22]. As a result of these findings, the combination is contraindicated in patients with a history of angioedema. It is also contraindicated during pregnancy, and if an ACE inhibitor has been administered within 36 hours of switching to the ARNI or if patients currently are receiving ACE inhibitors or have diabetes and are taking aliskerin [22].

4. New antidiabetic medications (liraglutide and empagliflozin)

Recent studies have shown beneficial effects of prototypes of two new groups of antidiabetic medications on cardiovascular events. Though results specifically for heart failure hospitalizations were significantly improved only with empagliflozin and did not reach statistical significance for liraglutide (studies of which had insufficient power to test the hypothesis that such events are prevented), there was clear numerical HF event reduction in patients with HFrEF with both drugs and, thus, inclusion in this chapter is appropriate.

Liraglutide is a glucagon-like peptide-1 (GLP-1) receptor agonist that enhances insulin secretion. One trial randomized 9340 patients with type 2 diabetes (HbA1c ≥ 7.0%) and underlying cardiovascular disease (CAD, cerebrovascular disease, PVD, CKD of stage 3 or greater, or chronic heart failure NYHA class II-III) to liraglutide or placebo on appropriate conventional background therapy [24]. The median time of exposure to liraglutide or placebo was 3.5 years. Death from cardiovascular causes (hazard ratio, 0.78 [95% CI, 0.66–0.93], p = 0.007), hospitalization for heart failure (hazard ratio, 0.87 [95% CI, 0.73–1.05], p = 0.14), and nonfatal myocardial infarction, nonfatal stroke, and death from any cause all were at least numerically lower in patients receiving liraglutide than placebo.

However, another far smaller double-blind, placebo-controlled randomized trial including 300 patients with type 2 diabetes and established HFrEF who were recently hospitalized did not reveal any beneficial effect of liraglutide [25]. The power of this trial was relatively low to find a significant difference if it existed, precluding firm conclusions about the role of liraglutide for HFrEF.

Another antidiabetic medication which may provide favorable effects on mortality and morbidity in patients with heart failure is empagliflozin, an inhibitor of the sodium glucose cotransporter-2 (SGLT-2), which enhances renal glucose excretion [26]. The placebo-controlled EMPA-REG trial assessed the effects of empagliflozin on cardiovascular morbidity and mortality in 7020 randomized patients with type 2 diabetes and established cardiovascular disease during a median follow-up of 3.1 years. Relative risk of cardiovascular death was reduced by 38% (3.7% with empagliflozin vs. 5.9% with placebo, hazard ratio, 0.62 [95% CI, 0.49–0.77], $p < 0.001$). Also, relative risk of hospitalization for heart failure was reduced by 35% (hazard ratio, 0.65 [95% CI, 0.50–0.85], p = 0.002). Death from any cause also was lower with empagliflozin (hazard ratio, 0.68 [95% CI, 0.57–0.82], $p < 0.001$).

5. Recent advances in device therapy

5.1. Left ventricular assist devices

Left ventricular assist devices (LVAD) are indwelling electromechanical pumps used to support cardiac function in patients with advanced heart failure. First successfully implanted in 1966 [27], such "first-generation" devices were limited by size and durability, were highly thrombogenic, and frequently complicated by infection. The mechanical design generally featured pulsatile displacement, analogous to the mechanism of pumping by the native heart [28]. More recent models have featured continuous flow with small rotating "impellers" moving blood forward. As a result, newer pumps are smaller and have no bearings (resulting in less mechanical wear and tear and greater durability than older models). Though generally introduced by thoracotomy and requiring a transcutaneous connection to an external generator, newer iterations are sufficiently slim such that they can be introduced percutaneously (the Impella device) via the femoral or axillary artery in the cardiac catheterization lab [29, 30]. Such percutaneously introduced devices have less pumping capacity than the more conventional models.

The effectiveness of LVAD was assessed in the Randomized Evaluation of Mechanical Assistance for the Treatment of Congestive Heart Failure (REMATCH) trial in 2001. The study involved 140 patients with advanced heart failure and contraindications to heart transplantation surgery. The trial revealed a LVAD associated 48% reduction in all-cause death (the primary endpoint) compared with medical therapy (relative risk, 0.52 [95% CI, 0.34–0.78], p = 0.001) [31].

In subsequent trials LVAD has reduced mortality and improved quality of life and functional capacity in patients with advanced heart failure. LVADs enhance total cardiac output by adding to that of the damaged native heart, potentially allowing myocardial recovery, particularly in patients with cardiogenic shock [30–34].

LVAD implantation currently is approved by FDA as a bridge to cardiac transplantation and also as "destination therapy" in selected patients for whom transplantation may not be feasible or possible [35].

Adverse events associated with LVAD use include thrombosis and thromboembolization (potentially leading to stroke), bleeding, and infection [31, 35].

5.2. Extracorporeal membrane oxygenators (ECMO)

ECMO devices enable extracorporeal circulation and physiologic gas exchange during acute respiratory and/or cardiorespiratory failure.

Two types of ECMO have been developed: veno-arterial extracorporeal membrane oxygenators (VA-ECMO) and veno-venous extracorporeal membrane oxygenators (VV-ECMO). FDA has approved application of VA-ECMO for short-term support in patients with refractory cardiogenic shock who have an underlying potentially reversible condition, acute onset refractory cardiogenic shock unresponsive to inotropes and/or intra-aortic balloon pump counterpulsation (IABP), and extracorporeal cardiopulmonary resuscitation (ECPR) [36].

Supporting data are case series from multiple countries [36–41]. In one study involving 45 patients with refractory cardiogenic shock, ECMO was associated with survival to hospital discharge in 29% (13/45) versus the expected total absence of survival without ECMO [40]. In another series, survival was achieved in 71% of patients with refractory cardiogenic failure during severe septic shock [41].

ECMO-associated adverse events include bleeding, infection, renal failure, liver failure, need for blood transfusion, hematuria, pulmonary complications, and need for thoracotomy [36].

5.3. Cardiac resynchronization therapy (CRT)

More than 20 years of research has established the role of CRT in patients with systolic heart failure and widened QRS complex. By the 1990s, a link emerged between electrical dyssynchrony and LV function, in which conduction disturbances result in an abnormally circuitous and lengthy conduction pathway, wasted work, and a reduction in cardiac output [42].

Intraventricular systolic dyssynchrony refers to lack of normal coordination in the timing of contraction between ventricular segments [43]. Dyssynchrony can be identified by multiple imaging techniques [44]. The prevalence of dyssynchrony is directly related to QRS duration and ventricular size and inversely related to left ventricular ejection fraction (LVEF) [43]. Prevalence of echocardiographically detectable dyssynchrony ranges from 27% in patients with QRS duration <120 ms, to 89% in those with QRS duration >150 ms [45].

CRT is effected by placing a pacemaker lead in each ventricle and setting the pacemaker generator to coordinate the stimuli to both ventricles, hence normalizing the contraction pattern. Mortality and morbidity (as well as symptoms) are consistently reduced (and LVEF and reverse remodeling improved) by CRT in patients with refractory HFrEF and prolonged QRS interval who are on optimal medical therapy [46–55].

CRT has been most clearly effective when QRS duration is abnormal, generally ≥150 ms with a left bundle branch block pattern, and when LVEF is ≤35%. However, recently, benefit for a wider range of patients has been explored. In BLOCK-HF, patients with HF symptoms, LVEF <50% and high degree AV block, who would otherwise be treated with RV pacing, were randomized to biventricular pacing versus RV pacing (patients who met the by then conventional more stringent CRT indications were excluded). CRT provided 26% reduction in the primary composite endpoint of total mortality, urgent HF care, or progression of increase in the LV end-systolic volume index [56].

In the randomized, double-blind LESSER-EARTH trial CRT was evaluated in patients with LVEF ≤35% and QRS <120 ms who failed to improve in clinical outcomes or LV reverse remodeling on conventional therapy. Importantly, dyssynchrony, determined by an imaging study, was not required for inclusion in the study. The trial was terminated prematurely due to futility and safety concerns, suggesting that CRT can worsen or provoke dyssynchrony in patients with little or no dyssynchrony [57].

EchoCRT carried this issue further by using rigorous imaging criteria to detect dyssynchrony among patients with QRS duration ≤130 ms, thus including those with nominally normal QRS duration (<120 ms) and those slightly higher, as well as HFrEF with LVEF ≤35%, LVED ≥55 mm and stable, guidelines-based pharmacological therapy [58]. Patients were randomized to CRT or no CRT. The study was stopped early due to futility, and death from cardiovascular causes was higher among patients who received CRT.

While normalizing conduction patterns alone can account for mechanical benefit, cellular and molecular alterations seem likely to contribute. Molecular mechanisms are not fully understood but, in experimental studies, CRT is associated with homogenization of stress kinase activity, potentially important in supporting contractile function, and reducing fibrosis [59].

CRT is also associated with decline in global apoptosis and enhanced cell-survival signaling [60, 61]. Biventricular pacing reduces interstitial remodeling [61]. TNF-α, which is not present in normal myocardium, stimulates fibrosis and apoptosis and contributes to the progression of heart failure by direct toxic effects [62] and is activated by mechanical stretch [63]. CRT lowers LV TNF-α after 6 months of therapy [61].

CRT also alters mitochondrial proteins [64] and upregulates β-1 receptors and adenylate cyclase activity [65] and partially ameliorates prolongation of the action potential duration (APD) selectively in the lateral wall [66].

http://dx.doi.org/10.5772/66284

Current AHA/ACC practice guideline* suggest application of CRT as follows [66]:

5.3.1. Class I indications:

1. CRT is indicated for patients who have LVEF of 35% or less, sinus rhythm, left bundle-branch block (LBBB) with a QRS duration of 150 ms or greater, and NYHA class II, III, or ambulatory IV symptoms on guideline-directed medical therapy (GDMT). (*Level of Evidence: A for NYHA class III/IV; Level of Evidence: B for NYHA class II*).

5.3.2. Class IIa indications:

1. CRT can be useful for patients who have LVEF ≤35%, sinus rhythm, a non-LBBB pattern with a QRS duration ≥150ms, and NYHA class III/ambulatory class IV symptoms on GDMT (*Level of Evidence: A*).

2. CRT can be useful for patients who have LVEF of 35% or less, sinus rhythm, LBBB with a QRS duration of 120–149 ms, and NYHA class II, III, or ambulatory IV symptoms on GDMT (*Level of Evidence: B*).

3. CRT can be useful in patients with AF and LVEF of 35% or less on GDMT if (a) the patient requires ventricular pacing or otherwise meets CRT criteria and (b) atrioventricular nodal ablation or pharmacological rate control will allow near 100% ventricular pacing with CRT (*Level of Evidence: B*).

4. CRT can be useful for patients on GDMT who have LVEF of 35% or less and are undergoing placement of a new or replacement device implantation with anticipated requirement for significant (>40%) ventricular pacing (*Level of Evidence: C*).

5.3.3. Class IIb indications

1. CRT may be considered for patients who have LVEF of 35% or less, sinus rhythm, a non-LBBB pattern with QRS duration of 120–149 ms, and NYHA class III/ambulatory class IV on GDMT (*Level of Evidence: B*).

2. CRT may be considered for patients who have LVEF of 35% or less, sinus rhythm, a non-LBBB pattern with a QRS duration of 150 ms or greater, and NYHA class II symptoms on GDMT (*Level of Evidence: B*).

3. CRT may be considered for patients who have LVEF of 30% or less, ischemic etiology of HF, sinus rhythm, LBBB with a QRS duration of 150 ms or greater, and NYHA class I symptoms on GDMT (*Level of Evidence: C*).

*These guidelines were published before BLOCK-HF and EchoCRT were published.

Use of CRT is associated with short- and long-term adverse effects [46–58]. Most commonly reported complications include coronary-sinus dissection/perforation, lead dislodgement, implantation site infection, hemo-/pneumothorax, pericardial effusion/pericarditis, hematoma, pacing failure, atrial fibrillation, inappropriate device stimulation of tissue, and DVT.

6. The future of therapy for heart failure

Future developments for heart failure therapy will focus on the major current deficiencies. For example, heart failure with preserved ejection fraction (HFpEF) is now known to account or approximately half the heart failure population, with the same 5-year survival rate as HFrEF. No life-prolonging or hospitalization reducing therapy now exists for patients with HFpEF though there has been a suggestion of possible benefit with spironolactone [67]. However, despite early hope with calcium channel blockers, there are no therapies specifically to prevent or reverse diastolic dysfunction or to prevent or reverse fibrosis, which may be important pathophysiological underpinnings of HFpEF (though these problems may be affected by therapies aiming at other cardiac functional targets). Both problems are under active drug development but no solutions have yet emerged. With regard to fibrosis, study in valve disease models [68] suggest that collagen, by far the predominant element of myocardial fibrous tissue, may not be the most appropriate target for preventive therapy, but that noncollagen elements, which can directly affect force transmission, may be the more appropriate targets. It is not clear whether this finding in regurgitant valve diseases, in which the myocardium is responding to extrinsic loading conditions, can be extrapolated to systolic heart failure in which intrinsic metabolic abnormalities are pathophysiologically most important. Moreover, though systolic function is importantly improved by several currently available therapies, drugs that specifically improve intrinsic myocardial contractility without countervailing adverse effects still are needed. One promising candidate is omecamtiv mecarbil [69], which enhances myosin cross-bridge formation and duration, thus increasing systolic ejection time, but without increasing oxygen utilization. Others may follow. Finally, a major adjunct to the therapies, themselves, is monitoring the effects of therapy to enable precise titration and maximize benefits [70]. Although beyond the scope of this chapter, it is clear that devices for remote monitoring are gaining ever greater impact on therapeutic decisions and will continue to be developed.

7. Conclusions

Therapy for heart failure and, specifically, for systolic heart failure (HFrEF), has progressed dramatically during the past 30 years. In addition to the use of diuretics to relieve volume overloading and associated symptoms, which already was established, five different groups of drugs and multiple devices have been developed and assessed in large randomized controlled clinical trials. The most recent of these developments, an f-current blocker to slow heart rate and a neprilysin blocker to enhance blood concentrations of several vasoactive substances, have added to the benefits on survival and hospitalization achieved by previously developed drugs that are still in use. At the same time, use of some drugs that were used conventionally before recent additions has diminished (e.g., digoxin), superseded by new developments. Innovations in therapeutic devices for heart failure also have moved rapidly though, over the past 5 years, the greatest advances have been in delineation of the appropriate application of existing devices. Nonetheless, 6 million Americans have heart failure as this is written and one million of them will be hospitalized this year. Therefore, research and

http://dx.doi.org/10.5772/66284

development of therapeutics remain importantly needed, most particularly focused in several areas. For example, no life-prolonging therapies yet have been identified for HFpEF (which affects half the heart failure population), no therapies specifically to mitigate diastolic dysfunction are available and no therapies specifically preventing myocardial fibrosis have been developed. Moreover, though systolic function is importantly improved by several currently available therapies, drugs that specifically improve intrinsic myocardial contractility without countervailing adverse effects still are needed. Thus, while the current therapeutic landscape reveals far more effective treatments than in the past, new research and development for heart failure therapeutics are greatly needed.

Author details

Oleg Yurevich[1] and Jeffrey S. Borer[2*]

*Address all correspondence to: jsborer1@gmail.com

1 Department of Medicine, SUNY Downstate Medical Center, Brooklyn, NY, USA

2 The Howard Gilman Institute for Heart Valve Diseases and The Schiavone Institute for Cardiovascular Translational Research, SUNY Downstate Medical Center, New York, NY, USA

References

[1] Mozzafarian D, Benjamin EJ, Go AS, Arnett DK, Blaha MJ, et al. Heart disease and stroke statistics – 2016 update: a report from the American Heart Association. *Circulation*. 2016; 133: e38–e360.

[2] Hall MJ, Levant S, DeFrances CJ. Hospitalization for congestive heart failure: United States, 2000–2010. *NCHS Data Brief* 2012; 108: 1–8.

[3] Kochanek KD, Murphy SL, Xu J, Tejada-Vera B. Deaths: Final Data for 2014. *Natl Vital Stat Rep* 2016; 65(4): 1–122.

[4] Official FDA website. FDA approves Corlanor to treat heart failure. http://www.fda.gov/NewsEvents/Newsroom/PressAnnouncements/ucm442978.htm. Accessed 8/29/2016.

[5] DiFrancesco D, Camm JA. Heart rate lowering by specific and selective I_f current inhibition with ivabradine: a new therapeutic perspective in cardiovascular disease. *Drugs* 2004; 64(16): 1757–1765.

[6] Ferrari R. Ivabradine: heart rate and left ventricular function. *Cardiology* 2014; 128: 226–230.

[7] Borer JS, Bohm M, Ford I, Komajda M, Tavazzi L, et al. Effect of ivabradine on recurrent hospitalization for worsening heart failure in patients with chronic systolic heart failure: the SHIFT Study. *Eur Heart J* 2012; 33: 2813–2820.

[8] Yancy CW, Jessup M, Bozkurt B, Butler J, Casey DE Jr, et al. Guidelines 2016 ACC/AHA/HFSA focused update on new pharmacological therapy for heart failure: an update of the 2013 ACCF/AHA guideline for the management of heart failure. A Report of the American College of Cardiology/American Heart Association Task Force on Clinical Practice Guidelines and the Heart Failure Society of America. *J Card Fail* 2016; 22: 659–669.

[9] Ferrari R, Ceconi C. Selective and specific I(f) inhibition with ivabradine: new perspectives for the treatment of cardiovascular disease. *Expert Rev Cardiovasc Ther* 2011; 9: 959–973.

[10] DiFrancesco D. The contribution of the 'pacemaker' current (I_f) to generation of spontaneous activity in rabbit sino-atrial node myocytes. *J Physiol* 1991; 434: 23–40.

[11] Swedberg K, Komajda M, Bohm M, Borer JS, Ford I, et al. Ivabradine and outcomes in chronic heart failure (SHIFT): a randomized placebo-controlled study. *Lancet* 2010; 11; 376: 875–885.

[12] Fang Y, Debunne M, Vercauteren M, Brakenhielm E, Richard V, et al. Heart rate reduction induced by the I_f current inhibitor ivabradine improves diastolic function and attenuates cardiac tissue hypoxia. *J Cardiovasc Pharmacol* 2012; 59: 260–267.

[13] Mancini GBJ, Howlett JG, Borer J, Liu PP, Mehra MR, et al. Pharmacologic options for the management of systolic heart failure: examining underlying mechanisms. *Can J Cardiol* 2015; 31: 1282–1292.

[14] Beltrame JF. Ivabradine and the SIGNIFY conundrum. *Eur Heart J* 2015; 36: 3297–3299.

[15] Official FDA website. http://www.accessdata.fda.gov/drugsatfda_docs/label/2015/206143Orig1s000lbl.pdf Accessed 8/30/2016.

[16] Savelieva I, Camm AJ. I_f inhibition with Ivabradine: electrophysiological effects and safety. *Drug Saf* 2008; 31: 95–107.

[17] Sargento L, Satendra M, Longo S, Lousada N, dos Reis RP. Heart rate reduction with ivabradine in patients with acute decompensated systolic heart failure. *Am J Cardiovasc Drugs* 2014; 14: 229–235.

[18] Pascual Izco M, Alonso Salinas GL, Sanmartin Fernandez M, Del Castillo Carnevalli H, Jimenez Mena M, et al. Clinical experience with ivabradine in acute heart failure. *Cardiology* 2016; 134: 372–374.

[19] Official FDA website. FDA approves new drug to treat heart failure. http://www.fda.gov/NewsEvents/Newsroom/PressAnnouncements/ucm453845.htm. Accessed 8/30/2016.

[20] Gayathiri K, Prabhavathi A, Tamilarasi R, Vimalavathini R, Kavimani S. Role of neprilysin in various diseases. *Int J of Pharmacol Res* 2014; 4: 91–94.

[21] Langenickel TH, Dole WP. Angiotensin receptor-neprilysin inhibition with LCZ696: a novel approach for the treatment of heart failure. *Drug Discov Today* 2012; 9: e131–139.

[22] Official FDA website. http://www.accessdata.fda.gov/drugsatfda_docs/label/2015/207620Orig1s000lbl.pdf. Accessed 8/30/2016.

[23] McMurray JJ, Packer M, Desai AS, Gong J, Lefkowitz MP, et al. Angiotensin-neprilysin inhibition versus enalapril in heart failure. *N Engl J Med*. 2014; 371: 993–1004.

[24] Marso SP, Daniels GH, Brown-Frandsen K, Kristensen P, Mann JF, et al. Liraglutide and cardiovascular outcomes in type 2 diabetes. *N Engl J Med*. 2016; 375(4): 311–322.

[25] Margulies KB, Hernandez AF, Redfield MM, Givertz MM, Oliveira GH, et al. Effects of liraglutide on clinical stability among patients with advanced heart failure and reduced ejection fraction: a randomized clinical trial. *JAMA*. 2016; 316(5): 500–508.

[26] Zinman B, Wanner C, Lachin JM, Fitchett D, Bluhmki E, et al. Empagliflozin, cardiovascular outcomes, and mortality in type 2 diabetes. *N Engl J Med*. 2015; 373(22): 2117–2128.

[27] Kirklin JK, Naftel DC. Mechanical circulatory support: registering a therapy in evolution. *Circ Heart Fail*. 2008; 1(3): 200–205.

[28] Fang JC. Rise of the machines — left ventricular assist devices as permanent therapy for advanced heart failure. *N Engl J Med* 2009; 361: 2282–2285.

[29] Lima B, Kale P, Gonzalez-Stawinski GV, Kuiper JJ, Carey S, et al. Effectiveness and safety of the Impella 5.0 as a bridge to cardiac transplantation or durable left ventricular assist device. *Am J Cardiol* 2016; 117: 1622–1628.

[30] Lauten A, Engström AE, Jung C. Percutaneous left-ventricular support with the Impella-2.5-sssist device in acute cardiogenic shock: results of the Impella-EURO-SHOCK-registry. *Circ Heart Fail* 2013; 6: 23–30.

[31] Rose EA, Gelijns AC, Moskowitz AJ, Heitjan DF, Stevenson LW, et al. Longs term use of a left ventricular assist device for end-stage heart failure. *N Engl J Med* 2001; 345: 1435–1443.

[32] Slaughter MS, Rogers JG, Milano CA, Russell SD, Conte JV, et al. Advanced heart failure treated with continuous-flow left ventricular assist device. *N Engl J Med* 2009; 361: 2241–2251.

[33] Seyfarth M, Sibbing D, Bauer I, Frohlich G, Bott-Flugel L, et al. A randomized clinical trial to evaluate the safety and efficacy of a percutaneous left ventricular assist device

versus intra-aortic balloon pumping for treatment of cardiogenic shock caused by myocardial infarction. *J Am Coll Cardiol* 2008; 52(19): 1584–1588.

[34] Griffith BP, Anderson MB, Samuels LE, Pae WE Jr, Naka Y, et al. The RECOVER I: a multicenter prospective study of Impella 5.0/LD for postcardiotomy circulatory support. *J Thorac Cardiovasc Surg* 2013; 145: 548–554.

[35] FDA website. Serious adverse events with implantable left ventricular assist devices (LVADs): FDA safety communication. http://www.fda.gov/MedicalDevices/Safety/AlertsandNotices/ucm457327.htm. Accessed 9/2/2016.

[36] FDA website. Classification of the membrane lung for long-term pulmonary support [Extracorporeal Membrane Oxygenator – ECMO (21 CFR 868.5610)]. http://www.fda.gov/downloads/AdvisoryCommittees/CommitteesMeetingMaterials/MedicalDevices/MedicalDevicesAdvisoryCommittee/CirculatorySystemDevicesPanel/UCM395652.pdf. Accessed 9/2/2016.

[37] Luo XJ, Wang W, Hu SS, Sun HS, Gao HW, et al. Extracorporeal membrane oxygenation for treatment of cardiac failure in adult patients. *Interact Cardiovasc Thorac Surg* 2009; 9(2): 296–300.

[38] Loforte A, Montalto A, Ranocchi F, Della Monica PL, Casali G, et al. Peripheral extracorporeal membrane oxygenation system as salvage treatment of patients with refractory cardiogenic shock: preliminary outcome evaluation. *Artif Organs* 2012; 36(3): E53–61.

[39] Formica F, Avalli L, Colagrande L, Ferro O, Greco G, et al. Extracorporeal membrane oxygenation to support adult patients with cardiac failure: predictive factors of 30-day mortality. *Interact Cardiovasc Thorac Surg* 2010; 10: 721–726.

[40] Bakhtiary F, Keller H, Dogan S, Dzemali O, Oezaslan F, et al. Venoarterial extracorporeal membrane oxygenation for treatment of cardiogenic shock: clinical experiences in 45 adult patients. *J Tthorac Cardiovasc Surg* 2008; 135(2): 382–388.

[41] Brechot N, Luyt CE, Schmidt M, Leprince P, Trouillet JL, et al. Venoarterial extracorporeal membrane oxygenation support for refractory cardiovascular dysfunction during severe bacterial septic shock. *Crit Care Med* 2013; 41(7): 1616–1626.

[42] Leyva F, Nisam S, Auricchio A. 20 years of cardiac resynchronization therapy. *J Am Coll Cardiol* 2014; 64: 1047–1058.

[43] Nagueh SF. Mechanical dyssynchrony in congestive heart failure. Diagnostic and therapeutic implications. *J Am Coll Cardiol*. 2008; 51(1): 18–22.

[44] Russo AM, Stainback RF, Bailey SR, Epstein AE, Heidenreich PA, et al. ACCF/HRS/AHA/ASE/HFSA/SCAI/SCCT/ SCMR 2013 Appropriate use criteria for implantable cardioverter-defibrillators and cardiac resynchronization therapy: a report of the American College of Cardiology Foundation appropriate use criteria task force, Heart Rhythm Society, American Heart Association, American Society

of Echocardiography, Heart Failure Society of America, Society for Cardiovascular Angiography and Interventions, Society of Cardiovascular Computed Tomography, and Society for Cardiovascular Magnetic Resonance. *J Am Coll Cardiol* 2013; 61: 1318–1368.

[45] Hawkins NM, Petrie MC, MacDonald MR, Hogg KJ, McMurray JJ. Selecting patients for cardiac resynchronization therapy: electrical or mechanical dyssynchrony? *Eur Heart J* 2006; 27: 1270–1281.

[46] Cazeau S, Leclercq C, Lavergne T, Walker S, Varma C, et al. Effects of multisite biventricular pacing in patients with heart failure and intraventricular conduction delay. *N Engl J Med* 2001; 344: 873–880.

[47] Auricchio A, Stellbrink C, Sack S, Block M, Vogt J, et al. Long-term clinical effect of hemodynamically optimized cardiac resynchronization therapy in patients with heart failure and ventricular conduction delay. *J Am Coll Cardiol* 2002; 39: 2026–2033.

[48] Abraham WT, Fisher WG, Smith AL, Delurgio DB, Leon AR, et al. Cardiac resynchronization in chronic heart failure. *N Engl J Med* 2002; 346: 1845–1853.

[49] Young JB, Abraham WT, Smith AL, Leon AR, Lieberman R, et al. Combined cardiac resynchronization and implantable cardioversion defibrillation in advanced chronic heart failure: the MIRACLE ICD Trial. *JAMA* 2003; 289: 2685–2694.

[50] Bristow MR, Saxon LA, Boehmer J, Krueger S, Kass DA, et al. Cardiac resynchronization therapy with or without an implantable defibrillator in advanced heart failure. *N Engl J Med* 2004; 350: 2140–2150.

[51] Cleland JG, Daubert JC, Erdmann E, Freemantle N, Gras D, et al. The effect of cardiac resynchronization on morbidity and mortality in heart failure. *N Engl J Med* 2005; 352: 1539–1549.

[52] Higgins SL, Hummel JD, Niazi IK, Giudici MC, Worley SJ, et al. Cardiac resynchronization therapy for the treatment of heart failure in patients with intraventricular conduction delay and malignant ventricular tachyarrhythmias. *J Am Coll Cardiol* 2003; 42:1454–1459.

[53] Abraham WT, Young JB, Leon AR, Adler S, Bank AJ, et al. Effects of cardiac resynchronization on disease progression in patients with left ventricular systolic dysfunction, an indication for an implan cardioverter-defibrillator, and mildly symptomatic chronic heart failure. *Circulation* 2004; 110: 2864–2868.

[54] Linde C, Abraham WT, Gold MR, St John Sutton M, Ghio S, et al. Randomized trial of cardiac resynchronization in mildly symptomatic heart failure patients and in asymptomatic patients with left ventricular dysfunction and previous heart failure symptoms. *J Am Coll Cardiol* 2008; 52: 1834–1843.

[55] Moss AJ, Hall WJ, Cannom DS, Klein H, Brown MW, et al. Cardiac-resynchronization therapy for the prevention of heart failure events. *N Engl J Med* 2009; 361: 1329–1338.

[56] Curtis AB, Worley SJ, Adamson PB, Chung ES, Niazi I, et al. Biventricular pacing for atrioventricular block and systolic dysfunction. *N Engl J Med* 2013; 368: 1585–1593.

[57] Thibault B, Harel F, Ducharme A, White M, Ellenbogen KA, et al. Cardiac resynchronization therapy in patients with heart failure and a QRS complex <120 milliseconds: the evaluation of resynchronization therapy for heart failure (LESSER-EARTH) trial. *Circulation* 2013; 127: 873–881.

[58] Ruschitzka F, Abraham WT, Singh JP, Bax JJ, Borer JS, et al. Cardiac-resynchronization therapy in heart failure with a narrow QRS complex. *N Engl J Med* 2013; 369: 1395–1405.

[59] Chakir K, Daya SK, Tunin RS, Helm RH, Byrne MJ, et al. Reversal of global apoptosis and regional stress kinase activation by cardiac resynchronization. *Circulation* 2008; 117:1369–1377.

[60] D'Ascia C, Cittadini A, Monti MG, Riccio G, Sacca L. Effects of biventricular pacing on interstitial remodelling, tumor necrosis factor-alpha expression, and apoptotic death in failing human myocardium. *Eur Heart J* 2006; 27: 201–206.

[61] Mann DL. Tumor necrosis factor-induced signal transduction and left ventricular remodeling. *J Card Fail* 2002; 8:379–386.

[62] Palmieri EA, Benincasa G, Di Rella F, Casaburi C, Monti MG, et al. Differential expression of TNF-α, IL-6, and IGF-1 by graded mechanical stress in normal rat myocardium. *Am J Physiol Heart Circ Physiol* 2002; 282: H926–H934.

[63] Agnetti G, Kaludercic N, Kane LA, Elliott ST, Guo Y, et al. Modulation of mitochondrial proteome and improved mitochondrial function by biventricular pacing of dyssynchronous failing hearts. *Circ Cardiovasc Genet* 2010; 3:78–87.

[64] Chakir K, Daya SK, Aiba T, Tunin RS, Dimaano VL, et al. Mechanisms of enhanced beta-adrenergic reserve from cardiac resynchronization therapy. *Circulation* 2009; 119: 1231–1240.

[65] Aiba T, Hesketh GG, Barth AS, Liu T, Daya S, et al. Electrophysiological consequences of dyssynchronous heart failure and its restoration by resynchronization therapy. *Circulation* 2009; 119: 1220–1230.

[66] Yancy CW, Jessup M, Bozkurt B, Butler J, Casey DE Jr, et al. 2013 ACCF/AHA guideline for the management of heart failure: a report of the American College of Cardiology Foundation/American Heart Association Task Force on practice guidelines. *Circulation*. 2013; 128: e240–e327.

[67] Pitt B, Pfeffer MA, Assmann SF, Boineau R, Anand IS, Claggett B, et al. Spironolactone for heart failure with preserved ejection fraction. *N Engl J Med* 2014; 370: 1383–1392.

[68] Borer JS, Truter SL, Herrold EM, Falcone DJ, Pena M, Carter JN, et al. Myocardial fibrosis in chronic aortic regurgitation: molecular and cellular response to volume overload. *Circulation* 2002; 105: 1837–1842.

http://dx.doi.org/10.5772/66284

[69] Teerlink JR. A novel approach to improve cardiac performance: cardiac myosin activators. *Heart Fail Rev*. 2009; 14: 289–298.

[70] Adamson PB, Abraham WT, Bourge RC, Costanzo MR, Hasan A, Yadav C, et al. Wireless pulmonary artery pressure monitoring guides management to reduce decompensation in heart failure with preserved ejection fraction. *Circ Heart Fail*. 2014; 7: 935–944.

Chapter 2

Sympathetic Blockade for Dysrhythmia Management in Heart Failure: Rationale and Therapeutic Progression to Intervention

Daryl I. Smith and Albert O. Duah

Additional information is available at the end of the chapter

http://dx.doi.org/10.5772/66517

Abstract

Continuous ganglionic blockade is being used increasingly to help manage ventricular tachydysrhythmias. The purpose of this chapter is to discuss the physiologic and anatomic basis of ventricular tachydysrhythmias in detail that are mediated by the sympathetic nervous system and to discuss appropriate indications for the use of sympathetic ganglion blocks. These blocks can be instituted as both destination and bridging therapeutic options to control these dysrhythmias. These blocks therefore have value in the heart failure patient population since they offer a means of controlling the dysrhythmias that can be devastating to an already compromised myocardium.

Keywords: electric storm, ventricular tachycardia, left cardiac sympathetic ganglion block, automatic implantable cardioverter-defibrillator, tachydysrhythmia

1. Introduction

1.1. Epidemiology of ventricular dysrhythmias in heart failure

Ventricular dysrhythmias present significant risk of death to patients suffering from heart failure resulting from valvular and ischemic diseases. Heart failure affects 6–10% of people over the age of 65 years [1]. Dysrhythmia in the setting of heart failure occurs at a reported incidence of 51% [2] and in studies it is reflected as causes of sudden death in patients diagnosed with congestive heart failure [3]. In otherwise healthy adults with frequent and complex ventricular ectopy, the long-term prognosis is similar to that of the healthy U.S. population and suggests no increased risk of death [4]. The implications are different in patients with depressed left ventricular function after an acute myocardial infarction in this setting, high ectopy, greater than 10 PVCs per hour, is a useful risk marker of fatal or near-fatal arrhythmias after myocardial infarction [5]. And in patients with CHF, nonsustained ventricular tachycardia (NSVT) is an independent marker for increased overall mortality rate and sudden death while the absence of NSVT and ventricular repetitive beats in a 24-h Holter indicates a low probability of sudden death [6].

It should be noted that VT and VF that occur in the setting of nonischemic dilated cardiomyopathies, i.e., not associated with acute ischemic heart disease, are the most common result of reentry involving a region of myocardial scar. These ventricular scars that result in reentrant VT also occur in idiopathic dilated cardiomyopathies, hypertrophic cardiomyopathy, infiltrative heart disease (e.g., sarcoidosis), and right ventricular dysplasia. While ischemic VT/VF may resolve as the ischemic insult is corrected [7], the ectopic foci in nonischemic dilated cardiomyopathy are more incessant since they involve reentrant circuits that are created over time and more difficult to treat since the circuits are larger in the hypertrophic myocardium [8]. This is also a component of the vicious circle that is created as the ventricle either dilates or hypertrophies. In this setting, changes occur at the molecular level. These create a milieu more conducive to the development of reentrant circuits. In addition, the dysrhythmias themselves can also cause hypertrophic remodeling of ventricular myocardium and the cycle is further sustained [8].

1.2. Electrical storm

Electric storm is a variant of ventricular tachydysrhythmias (tachycardia or fibrillation) in which three or more sustained episodes of these dysrhythmias, or consequent shocks from an automatic implantable cardioverter-defibrillator occur within in a 24-h period. The syndrome typically manifests during acute myocardial infarction, in patients who have structural heart disease such as hypertrophic cardiomyopathy, in patients who have an implantable cardioverter-defibrillator, or in individuals suffering from an inherited dysrhythmic syndrome [9].

1.3. Description of strategies to control ventricular dysrhythmias

Efforts to control these dysrhythmias begin with pharmacologic interventions, progress to implantable devices to control or eradicate aberrant rhythms, followed by ablative techniques to locate and deactivate anatomic sites of dysrhythmogenesis, and frequently end in attempts to interrupt the sites of adrenergic innervation to the myocardium. The purpose of this chapter is to review these techniques with emphasis upon the recent work on left sympathetic cardiac denervation.

2. Review of the neuroanatomy and physiology of sympathetic cardiac innervation

The optimal activity of the heart is regulated by the central nervous system through the autonomic innervation of the heart. Cardiac dysrhythmias and sudden cardiac death may be a result of dysfunction of this cardiac activity-regulating circuitry [10]. Sympathetic and parasympathetic branches of the cardiac autonomic nervous system (ANS) work primarily through actions of cardiac pacemaker tissue to modulate heart rate and conduction velocity.

2.1. Sympathetic and parasympathetic innervation

Parasympathetic neurons receive preganglionic inputs from the vagus. The parasympathetic neurons synapse at ganglia located directly on the heart. These neurons have their cell bodies within the cardiac ganglia, arranged in discrete locations within the atrial epicardium, in plexi along the walls of the major cardiac vessels, and within the ventricular wall [11].

2.2. Neurotransmitters of the cardiac autonomic nervous system

The primary neurotransmitter in these cardiac parasympathetic ganglionic neurons is acetylcholine; however, vasoactive intestinal polypeptide (VIP) and nitrous oxide may also be coreleased from parasympathetic terminals [12, 13]. The sympathetic neurons essentially use norepinephrine as their principal neurotransmitter, although other neurotransmitters, such as neuropeptide Y (NPY) and galanin, are coreleased from sympathetic terminals [14, 15]. Among other functions, NPY and galanin decrease acetylcholine release from adjacent parasympathetic terminals.

2.3. Anatomy of the cardiac autonomic nervous system

The preganglionic sympathetic fibers are located in the lateral column of the spinal cord travel along nerves and the adventitia of blood vessels to form three cervical ganglia and the first three or four thoracic ganglia [16]. Sympathetic cardiac neurons have their cell bodies within the three cervical ganglia, the superior cervical ganglion, the middle cervical ganglion, and the inferior cervical ganglion. The cardiac branches of the superior cervical ganglion (located in front of the C2 and C3 vertebrae) originate in the inferior sector of the ganglion and travel down the carotid and in front of the large muscles of the neck. The middle cervical ganglion located at the level of C6 and near the inferior thyroid artery has a cardiac branch that arises independently or appears after synapse with the inferior cervical ganglion. On the right side, it constitutes the dorsal part of the cardiac plexus and on the left side it converges at the deep part of the cardiac plexus. The inferior cervical ganglion is located between the base of the transverse process of the last cervical vertebra and the first rib, on the medial side of the costocervical artery. The cardiac branch of the inferior cervical ganglion converges with the recurrent nerve and with a branch of the medium cervical nerve before joining the deep part of the cardiac plexus [16]. This combination of inferior and middle cervical ganglion neurons constitutes the paravertebral stellate ganglion. Ninety-two percent of retrograde-labeled nerves from the heart have their origins in the thoracic paravertebral ganglia [17, 18]. Thus, postganglionic cardiac sympathetic neurons have their cell bodies primarily in these ganglia.

Sympathetic efferent nerves are also present in the myocytes of the atrial and ventricular muscle and can thereby influence force of contraction and relaxation. For control of heart rate, the physical proximity of postganglionic cardiac parasympathetic and sympathetic axons to pacemaker regions permits the formation of synapses and modulation of pacemaker function, through either acetylcholine inhibition of norepinephrine release or vice versa [11]. Parasympathetic effects on the sinus node predominate over sympathetic effects despite mutual modulation. The intrinsic cardiac nervous system provides an additional level of complexity within peripheral autonomic interactions. Within cardiac ganglia, integration of parasympathetic, sensory, and sympathetic inputs by way of local circuit neurons occurs. This level of integration is critical for local regulation of heart rate on a beat-to-beat basis via rapid temporal reflexes [11].

2.4. Theories of ventricular dysrhythmia generation

Aside from intraganglionic cross talk, interganglionic connections and descending inputs play a pivotal role in this regulation of heart rate on a beat-to-beat basis [19, 20]. Neuronal connections between sympathetic nerves and parasympathetic neurons also mediate prejunctional autonomic interactions within the cardiac ganglia [21]. For example, ablation of the right atrial ganglion plexus attenuates vagal bradycardia while retaining vagal inhibition of sympathetic function [21, 22]. Armour et al. demonstrated neurons within the ganglia that do not project their axons beyond the ganglion (local circuit neurons) constitute a majority of the neurons in the mammalian cardiac ganglion [21, 23]. Cardiac ganglia therefore represent an important site for peripheral autonomic interactions.

The concept of sympathetic over activity, usually accompanied by reduced parasympathetic activity and heart rate variability, is increasingly recognized as a feature in the pathogenesis of a number of cardiovascular diseases [11]. Chen et al. postulated the nerve-sprouting hypothesis of sudden cardiac death which links nerve sprouting and electrical remodeling [24]. A number of studies have demonstrated the presence of aberrant sympathetic or parasympathetic outgrowth in human and canine hearts with atrial fibrillation [11]. Studies have demonstrated that ectopic or reentrant activity occurs at locations where autonomic fibers aggregate, such as the ligament of Marshall [11]. This has made ablation therapy, or localized cardiac denervation or block, a common option for reversing atrial or ventricular fibrillation episodes [11]. Foci for ventricular arrhythmia generation are much more likely to develop in areas where electrical signaling is discontinuous, such as an area of fibrosis, or where the myocardium is hypersensitive to catecholamines due to functional or pathological denervation. Consequently, the effectiveness of these therapies has been affected by the residual presence of scar tissue or fibrosis that will continue to serve as a substrate for arrhythmia generation. It has been demonstrated that robust and prolonged sympathetic hyperinnervation also occurs in cardiac-projecting stellate ganglia after acute myocardial infarction [11].

3. Pharmacologic management of ventricular dysrhythmias

3.1. Classes of cardiac drugs and mechanisms of action

Pharmacologic management is the initial treatment option for ventricular tachyarrhythmias. Given that heart failure is a state with high catecholamine levels, drugs that act through the decrease of this effect are of significant benefit [25]. The antisympathetic effect of beta blockers, for example, has been shown to be protective especially during myocardial ischemia by increasing the threshold for ventricular fibrillation and by reducing the catecholamine-induced influx of calcium into cells during the repolarization phase of the cardiac action potential [26–28]. These protective effects are not absolute and may be lost with increase in sympathetic activity that cannot be compensated [29, 30]. A brief summary of the classes of cardiac drugs and their suspected mechanisms of action are shown in **Tables 1** and **2**.

Class	Agent studied	Effect on mortality in CHF
I	Propafenone [31] Flecainide [31] Encainide [31] Moricizine [32]	Increase in death rate noted [31, 32]
II	Metoprolol [33] Carvedilol [34] Bisoprolol [35]	Mortality decreased [33–35]
III	Amiodarone [6, 36–39] Dofetilide [40]	No demonstrable improvement in survival [6, 36, 37] Possibly mortality reduction in nonischemic cardiomyopathy [38] No improvement in mortality [40]
IV	Verapamil [41–43]	Does not affect VT caused by reentry and catecholamine-sensitivity [41, 43] Not studied in patients with VT/VF and CHF

Table 1. Summary of drug class application and efficacy in the setting of ventricular tachycardia/fibrillation and heart failure.

We should elaborate here some of the current considerations of increased mortality associated with amiodarone therapy. This increased mortality with amiodarone exists in the setting of acute myocardial infarction and heart failure. Thomas et al. examined mortality related to amiodarone therapy at consecutive periods following acute myocardial infarction with heart failure and/or left ventricular systolic dysfunction. The postacute MI time periods studied were days 1–16, 17–45, 46–198, and 199–1096. The authors found significant increases in mortality in 3 of the 4 periods (days 1–16, 17–45, and 199–1096). The group concluded that the use of amiodarone was associated with excess early and late all-cause mortality as well as cardiac-related mortality [44].

In another study examining amiodarone-related mortality, Torp-Pedersen et al. examined 155 of 1466 NYHA class II patients who received amiodarone at baseline and 209 of 1563 NYHA class III or IV patients who received amiodarone at baseline. Sixty-six percent of all the patients who received amiodarone were followed for 4 years. The authors found that 38.7–58.9% of patients receiving amiodarone in NYHA class II and class III–IV, respectively, died, versus 26.2–43.3% not receiving amiodarone ($p < 0.001$). They concluded that amiodarone was associated with an increased risk of death. This risk was independent of functional class [45].

	Phase of cardiac action potential affected
Class I (sodium channel blockers) Ia (quinidine, procainamide)	Phase 0 Na^+ channel blockers; (intermediate association/ dissociation)
Ib (lidocaine, phenytoin)	Phase 0 Na^+ channel blockers (fast association/ dissociation)
Ic (flecanide, propafenone)	Phase 0 Na^+ channel blockers (slow association/ dissociation)
Class II (beta blockers) Propranolol, metoprolol	Phase 4 (propranolol also shows some class I action); Metoprolol is a selective beta1-adrenergic receptor blocker that decreases the automaticity of contractions
Class III (potassium channel blockers) Amiodarone, sotalol	Phases 1, 2, 4 (sotalol is also a beta blocker; amiodarone has class I, II, III, and IV activity, and is currently the drug of choice for acute, hemodynamically unstable ventricular tachycardia that is refractory to other antiarrhythmic agents)
Class IV (calcium channel blockers) Verapamil, diltiazem	Phase 2 Ca channel blockers
Class V Adenosine, digoxin	Unknown mechanisms (direct nodal inhibition)

Table 2. Summary cardiac drug classes and the cardiac action potential phase affected.

3.2. Molecular bases of class II (β-blockers) cardiac drugs

As noted above, congestive heart failure is a condition associated with elevated levels of serum catecholamines and with all of the well-described sequelae of an increase in sympathetic agonism. The mechanism of these effects is well described and pertinent to the understanding of the specific interventions discussed in this chapter and warrants review in order to knowledgeably address the treatment plan for ventricular tachyarrhythmias in the setting of congestive heart failure. When activated, the sympathetic fibers release norepinephrine, which binds to the transmembrane, GCPR-class β-adrenergic receptors. The receptors generate membrane-associated adenylyl cyclases (AC) which increases the membrane levels of cyclic adenylyl monophosphate (cAMP). This is transported across the cell membrane where it activates a number of intracellular effectors [46]. These effectors include phosphodiesterase (PDE), cAMP-dependent guanine nucleotide exchange factors (Epacs), [47–49] and protein kinase A (PKA). All of these play a role in the pathophysiology of heart failure with PDE and the Epacs acting on a cellular and genetic level in the pathologic remodeling of the hypertrophic myocardium [50, 51]. All of these effectors are activated by the binding of agonists to the β-receptor and each are tethered to their downstream targets by the A-kinase anchoring protein (AKAP) making them available for phosphorylation and subsequent deactivation or offset [52, 53]. In the case of protein kinase A which is the third and channel-specific effector, we find that in its activated form the kinase phosphorylates L-type calcium channels. This activation causes increased calcium entry into the cells. The calcium ion channel has an equilibrium that is above the resting potential which results in depolarization when this potential is restored. In myocytes, the L-channel effector interaction increases membrane Ca^{2+} currents and Ca^{2+} release from the sarcoplasmic reticulum (SR) during each action potential, resulting in increased force production. In addition, Ca^{2+} reuptake into the SR is enhanced, thereby accelerating relaxation. Together, the inotropic (contractile) and lusitropic (relaxation) effects of sympathetic stimulation result in increased stroke volume [54]. In the sino-atrial node, activation of β-adrenergic receptors increases the heart rate via effector binding at both L-type and T-type channels. In this setting, as in the myocytes, an increase in cellular calcium entry, a more rapid return to the above-threshold resting potential, and subsequent depolarization occur when this potential is restored [55].

It is important to note that the tethering of the kinase to the calcium channel also makes it susceptible to rapid offset once the β-adrenergic stimulation has been removed.

The effectiveness of pharmacologic interventions in the treatment of ventricular dysrhythmias in the setting of heart failure is not absolute. In the event of treatment failure with the initial pharmacologic approach, more invasive techniques may be employed. Currently, the literature supports the combination of electrophysiologically guided antiarrhythmic therapy with implantable defibrillators to reduce the risk of sudden death in high-risk patients with coronary disease. However, in this setting, antiarrhythmic drugs alone are not recommended [56]. In the following section, we discuss implantable devices, the next level step in the treatment of CHF-related dysrhythmia.

4. Implantable devices and management of ventricular dysrhythmias

4.1. Automatic implantable cardiodefibrillators (AICD) and cardiac resynchronization therapy (CRT)

In a 2010 study, Tang et al. found that in patients with NYHA class II or III CHF and LVEF of 35% or less (one of the objective criteria of heart failure), amiodarone had no favorable effect on survival, whereas single-lead, shock-only AICD therapy reduced overall mortality by 23%. The median LVEF in patients was 25%; 70% were in NYHA class II, and 30% were in class III CHF. The cause of CHF was ischemic in 52% and nonischemic in 48%. AICD therapy was associated with a decreased risk of death of 23% and an absolute decrease in mortality of 7.2% at 5 years in the overall population. Results did not vary according to either ischemic or nonischemic causes of CHF, but they did vary according to the NYHA class [57].

AICD therapy can be used alone as the primary, preventive treatment of recurrent ventricular tachyarrhythmias in order to reduce the total mortality from sudden cardiac death.

In this chapter, we will discuss only the indications for use of ICD in patients with nonischemic heart failure (symptomatic with LVEF ≤ 35) as per guidelines set forth by the American College of Cardiology, the American College of Cardiology Foundation, the American Heart Association, the Heart Rhythm Society, and the New York Heart Association [58–62]. In this clinical setting, we find some variation in the specific aspects of recommendations for the use of ICD. It is important to note the points of intersection of these recommendations with respect to the use of ICD in heart failure. All guidelines recommend ICD placement when nonischemic cardiomyopathy and heart failure coexist. Heart failure is defined objectively in the guidelines as a left ventricular ejection fraction (LVEF) less than 40% and in most of the studies less than 35%. The dysrhythmias for which the ICD is recommended in the heart failure setting are ventricular fibrillation, hemodynamically unstable ventricular tachycardias, ventricular tachycardia with syncope, and sustained ventricular tachycardia. Most of the guidelines indicate that ICD treatment should be used in conjunction with optimized medical therapy, and in patients who have a reasonable expectation of meaningful survival for more than 1 year (**Table 3**) [59].

Cardiac resynchronization therapy (CRT) is an alternate, more advanced form of device therapy which is indicated for patients with systolic heart failure with quick response service (QRS) duration above 120 ms. The prolonged QRS is often associated with atrioventricular conduction delay and has been described as a risk factor for both all-cause cardiac death as well as sudden cardiac death (SCD) in patients with dilated cardiomyopathy [63]. CRT results in significant improvement in patients who have moderate-to-severe heart failure (NYHA class III/IV).

CRT allows biventricular pacing and was first described for use in congestive heart failure in 1994 [64]. In addition to improving cardiac output by stabilizing contraction and ejection patterns, it also has been shown to reverse pathologic remodeling of the hypertrophic ventricles in patients with congestive heart failure. This improvement is based upon the restoration of electrical synchrony with CRT which improves global cardiac function, energetics, and molecular and cellular phenotype [65].

The procedure for establishing a CRT pacing is more complex than that required to place an AICD alone. The technique involves insertion of a right ventricular endocardial lead via cephalic or subclavian vein approach as accomplished in AICD implantation. CRT also utilizes the insertion of a left ventricular lead which is also placed with access to the left ventricle obtained through cephalic or subclavian vein approaches. The most commonly used technique for left ventricular lead placement is to access the chamber via a coronary sinus tributary to reach the left ventricular free wall [66–68]. Khan et al. reported that the targeted approach to LV lead placement in CRT results in reversal of pathologic LV remodeling, clinical status, and the improvement of patient outcomes at long term follow-up as determined by the endpoints of combined death and heart failure-related hospital admissions [68].

There exists a modification of CRT in which a defibrillator function is added (CRT-D) and a number of studies have compared the two modalities. A systematic review of the literature compared CRT and CRT-D revealed a decrease in all-cause death rate after 1 year with CRT-D. These differences were noted in all-cause death rate after 1 year and cardiac death in the patients with LV impairment. The authors indicated that larger, randomized studies needed to be performed. In the review, subgroup analysis described four studies that addressed sudden cardiac death and revealed an odds ratio of 0.20 at the 95% confidence level in the longest follow-up period; and further subgroup analysis demonstrated superiority of the CRT-D group as an OR of 0.18 at the shorter follow period of >1 year [69].

http://dx.doi.org/10.5772/66517

Clinical setting (myocardial derangement)	Left ventricular ejection fraction (LVEF)	Dysrhythmia	Prior optimization of medical treatment	ICD therapy	Expectation for survival	Type of prevention
CHF (by LVEF) [62]	≤40	VF or hemodynamically unstable VT; VT with syncope	N/A	Recommended	≥1 year	Secondary
Nonischemic dilated cardiomyopathy [62]	N/A but significant LV dysfunction	Sustained VT or VF	Receiving chronic optimal medical therapy	Should be implanted	≥1 year	N/A
Non-ischemic heart disease, NYHA class II or III [62]	≤30–35%	N/A	Receiving chronic optimal medical therapy	Recommended	≥1 year (with good functional status)	Primary
Nonischemic dilated cardiomyopathy, NYHA class II or III [58]	≤35%	N/A	N/A	Indicated	N/A	N/A
Nonischemic dilated cardiomyopathy (or ischemic heart disease > 40 days post MI) [58]	≤35%	N/A	Receiving chronic, guideline-directed	Recommended	≥1 year (meaningful survival)	Primary

Table 3. Summary of the clinical recommendations of the use of ICD therapy in patients with nonischemic cardiomyopathy.

In 2013, Gold et al. examined 419 patients from the REVERSE (*Re*synchronization *reverses* *re*modeling in *s*ystolic left ventricular dysfunction) trial, a multicenter, randomized trial of patients suffering from CHF who were randomized to active CRT, CRT-pacemaker, and CRT-defibrillator groups. At 12 months of CRT, no significant difference in the study of primary outcomes was noted, however, at long-term follow-up which occurred over the ensuing 5 years the group found improved survival in patients with heart failure [70].

In 2004, Bristow et al. compared CRT with and without an implantable defibrillator in advanced chronic heart failure. They evaluated 1520 patients of NYHA class III and IV heart failure due to ischemic and nonischemic cardiomyopathy. They examined a composite primary endpoint which consisted of time to death or hospitalization for any cause. The study revealed that CRT-P and CRT-D when compared to optimal medical therapy, each decreased the risk of the primary end point with hazard ratios of 0.81 ($p = 0.014$), and 0.80 ($p = 0.01$) respectively. The risk of the combined end point of death and time to hospitalization for heart failure was reduced by 34% in the pacemaker group ($p < 0.002$) and 40% in the pacemaker-defibrillator group ($p < 0.001$) [71].

A decade later, Kutyifa et al. compared the effect of CRT-D with CRT-P in a high volume single-center setting. In this study, 693 CRT-P devices and 429 CRT-D devices were implanted in patients with mean LVEF = 28.2 (±7.4%) and 27.6 (± 6.4%), respectively. The median follow-up period was 28 months. In the CRT-P group, 250 patients died compared with 129 patients in the CRT-D group for percentage mortalities of 36% and 30, respectively. This was not statistically significant ($p = 0.894$). In patients with ischemic cardiomyopathy, CRT-D treatment was associated with a 30% risk reduction in all-cause mortality when compared with an implanted CRT-P ($p = 0.03$). In nonischemic patients no benefit was seen in CRT-D over CRT-P ($p = 0.15$) [72]. Currently, there are no large scale studies that directly compare the efficacy or safety of CRT versus AICD.

It should be noted that in the setting of atrial fibrillation, a recent meta-analysis has sought to compare radiofrequency ablation versus antiarrhythmic drug therapy examining as primary outcomes of quality of life, morbidity, and mortality. The authors concluded from their data that RFA demonstrates an early but nonsustained superiority over antiarrhythmic drug therapy for the improvement of quality of life in patients with atrial fibrillation. Whether this can be extrapolated to ventricular tachyarrhythmias remains to be determined [73].

In an earlier single center study, Morillo et al. examined RFA versus antiarrhythmic drugs as a first line treatment of paroxysmal atrial fibrillation. These authors concluded that among patients with paroxysmal AF without previous antiarrhythmic drug treatment, ablation compared with antiarrhythmic drugs (AAD) resulted in a lower rate of recurrent atrial tachyarrhythmias at 2 years. Recurrence was documented in approximately 50% of patients. Again, while the superiority of RFA over AAD is asserted in this work, the extrapolation to the setting of ventricular tachyarrhythmias cannot be assumed until similar studies in this condition are conducted [74].

4.2. Ablation therapy

Unifocal ventricular ectopic beats (VEBs) are frequently seen in clinical practice and are usually benign in nature. In patients with heart disease, however, there is a risk of sudden cardiac death from malignant ventricular arrhythmias if the VEBs persist and are frequent. As discussed in the earlier section, β-blockers may be used for symptom control in patients with impaired systolic function and/or heart failure if there is a significant risk of sudden cardiac death from VEB-triggered tachyarrhythmias. In unifocal VEBs arising from the right ventricular outflow tract in particular, catheter ablation may be considered in some patients as an adjunctive treatment [75].

In 1995, Zhu described the successful use of intracardiac mapping and radiofrequency catheter ablation to eliminate drug-refractory monomorphic VEBs in severely symptomatic patients. They examined 10 patients who met the selection criteria of frequent monomorphic ventricular ectopic activity-related symptoms. These symptoms were frequent episodes of palpitation, fatigue, dyspnea, and light-headedness. The symptoms persisted for a mean of 10 years (range 1–29). The criteria also included the inability to tolerate, or treatment failure with, at least three anti-arrhythmic drugs; no evidence of other cardiac arrhythmias (which differs from many other intervention criteria); and the absence of electrolyte abnormalities. All patients showed frequent ectopy with a mean of 17 (±11) VEB/min; or mean 1065 (±631) VEB/h with a range of 280–2094 VEB/h. The technique for ablation involved detailed mapping of the ventricular ectopic focus followed by definition of the earliest site of endocardial activation during spontaneous ventricular ectopic activity. Pace mapping was performed at the endocardial sites showing early activation (local endocardial potentials earlier than the surface QRS recording) during ventricular ectopic activity.

In their conclusion, the authors recommended the use of radiofrequency catheter ablation based upon the high success rate, the absence of complications, and resolution of symptoms related to frequent ventricular ectopic activity. The authors reemphasized that the ectopic activity target was monomorphic in nature and drug-resistant. The limitation of this work was the small sample size, the lack of true controls, and the inability to create true blinding, and fact that the data were collected from several centers without a standardized protocol. Based upon these data, with appropriate selection of patients, optimal clinical outcomes can be achieved.

The safety and efficacy of radiofrequency catheter ablation for ventricular tachycardia was evaluated by Calkins et al. in a prospective multicenter study. The work asserted that catheter ablation of VT associated with structural heart disease is more difficult than ablation of idiopathic VT and reasoned that the larger size of responsible reentrant circuits in hypertrophic hearts made complete ablation a greater challenge. In their study, 146 patients with structural heart disease and ventricular tachycardia underwent an attempt at ablation. They were followed at 243 (±153) days. In 75% of the patients, all mappable VTs were eliminated. Fifty-seven patients (41%) had no VT of any type. Twelve patients (8%) experienced a major complication which the authors stated was a "moderate" incidence [8]. The major complications were four strokes or transient ischemic attacks, four episodes of pericardial tamponade; complete heart block in two patients; and myocardial infarction and aortic valve injury in one patient. The authors also describe four procedure-related deaths. Three of the four deaths occurred in patients with ischemic cardiomyopathy. In this group, one death was the result of a 99% occlusion of the left main coronary artery. This was caused by coronary artery emboli that ultimately lead to cardiogenic shock and death. In a second death, (also in a patient with severe ischemic cardiomyopathy), the initial insult was cardiac tamponade which was thought to be the result of the use of a transseptal approach to advance the ablation catheter into the left ventricle. Following pericardiocentesis the patient developed pneumonia, progressive heart failure, and death 1 week later. A third death was attributed to a cerebrovascular accident that progressed to herniation and death. The fourth death was in a patient with ischemic cardiomyopathy with an LVEF = 15%, moderate mitral valve regurgitation and mild aortic insufficiency. The aortic insufficiency worsened after ablation and the patient underwent a previously planned coronary artery bypass graft. An aortic valve replacement and a mitral valve annuloplasty were also performed. Surgical exposure revealed that the aortic valve was noted to be friable with a tear attributed to the ablation catheter. The patient succumbed to cardiogenic shock on the first postoperative day [8].

Long-term survival analyses in this study revealed 22 deaths that were not procedure-related. Of these, two deaths were attributed to noncardiac causes (cancer and chronic obstructive pulmonary disease). Sixteen were classified as cardiac nondysrythmic deaths (e.g., pump failure) and four deaths were thought to be secondary to ventricular dysrhythmia. The overall 1 year survival postprocedure in the study was reported to be 75% [8].

The authors also report in this study that 54% of patients remained free of VT during follow-up. It should be noted that in this study, Calkins et al. reported the postablation occurrence of any VT, which resulted in an ICD discharge as having a recurrence whether the VT was the monomorphic VT targeted by the ablation or whether it was a polymorphic VT that may have been thought unrelated. This was an admirable, effective, and purposeful attempt to remove possible bias [8].

There is considerably less data regarding catheter ablation in the setting of nonischemic cardiomyopathy. Kottkamp et al. examined radio-frequency catheter ablation in eight patients with idiopathic dilated cardiomyopathy. The inclusion criteria for ablation were incessant VT (n = 4); frequent recurrent VT, reproducibly inducible with programmed electrical stimulation (n = 5). Of the eight patients examined in this study, three had suffered "aborted sudden cardiac death" and two had experienced syncope [76]. Two patients were dependent on mechanical ventilation and were catecholamine dependent for circulatory support at the time of attempted ablation. Following the ablation, the authors report that six of the nine target VTs were rendered noninducible. In six patients, VTs with ECG morphologies other than the target VTs were inducible following RF catheter ablation. The authors concluded that RF catheter ablation in a select group of patients with idiopathic dilated cardiomyopathy is feasible with a higher success rate in patients with incessant VT and a moderate success rate in patients with chronic VT. It should be noted that in contrast to electrical storm (defined as multiple recurrences of ventricular arrhythmias over a short period of time) [77], incessant VT is defined as hemodynamically stable VT which persists for longer than 1 h [77].

5. Sympathetic denervation

5.1. History

The use of sympathetic denervation to treat disease is not new. The earliest reported observations of possible beneficial effects of resection of sympathetic nerves were written by Francois

Frank who examined the intervention in Graves' disease (maladie de Basedow), epilepsy, glaucoma, and developmental delay. He also suggested in the work that angina might be treated by this resection as well [78]. In 1916, Jonescu used surgical left stellate ganglionectomy to successfully treat a patient with incapacitating angina and cardiac dysrhythmias [79, 80].

The role of stellate ganglion interruption alone was brought into question by Danielopolu who stated that the maneuver would likely not control anginal events, and advocated more extensive denervation which would include C5 to T6 [81]. Interestingly, the advent and efficacy of β-blockade therapy relegated sympathectomy to a less prominent role in management of heart disease [80]. The slow resurgence of sympathectomy came on the heels of a case report by Estes and Izlar in 2014 in which they described a patient with a refractory case of recurrent ventricular tachycardia. They performed bilateral cardiac sympathectomy and noted that after the operation there was normalization of a prolonged QRS conduction time [82]. In 1968, Zipes et al. presented a case of a patient with recurrent paroxysmal ventricular tachycardia/fibrillation and reviewed three modes of therapy used to obtain complete suppression of the ectopic ventricular foci: pacing, cardiac sympathetic denervation, and β-adrenal blockade [83]. Subsequent animal research by Fowlis et al. emphasized work with acute myocardial ischemia in awake, canine models. In this study, bilateral cardiac sympathetic denervation was performed and the dogs underwent two-stage left coronary artery ligation 6 months following the sympathectomy. The group reported 22% mortality from ventricular fibrillation at 15 min in postsympathectomy animals compared to 52% in control animals. They noticed a similar trend at 24 h where they found 44% VF-related mortality and 65% VF-related mortality in the postsympathectomy and control groups, respectively. The study also revealed a significantly greater percentage increase in the sinus cardiac rate 1 min after LCA occlusion in control animals versus postsympathectomy animals. Later onset ventricular dysrhythmias were noted as well as a lesser incidence of ventricular premature beats. They concluded that sympathectomy imparted a protective effect from VF following experimental coronary occlusion in conscious animals [84].

5.2. Experimental foundation of sympathetic denervation

The experimental foundation for sympathetic denervation in treating ventricular tachyarrhythmias was further established in a study by Schwartz and Stone in 1980 in which they established the prevention of ventricular fibrillation by acute myocardial ischemia in a conscious canine model following sympathetic denervation [85]. In the human model, an ebb and flow existed in clinical confidence in left cardiac sympathetic blockade. This was caused by a perceived lack of reliable shortening of a prolonged QT interval in patients affected by syndromes that involved this phenomenon and directly followed the landmark work of Moss and McDonald in 1971 [86]. The misconception was based upon the belief that a pharmacologic blockade of the left stellate ganglion would reliably recreate the physiologic effect of the technique used by Moss which resulted in Horner's syndrome. Horner's syndrome, which was classically used as a marker of an effective sympathetic blockade, does not ensure that the lower fibers of the stellate ganglion or the thoracic cardiac have been blocked. Currently, there remains a lack of rigorous clinical data. Treatment, then, is predicated upon extrapolation from animal models and a growing number of clinical anecdotes and case series that are suggestive of the efficacy and safety of the technique in humans.

One of the few studies to critically examine the relationship between sympathetic hypersensitivity as a clinical trigger of life-threatening dysrhythmias and the use of sympathetic denervation as a viable intervention was performed by Schwartz et al. [87]. In this placebo controlled, multicenter study, the efficacies of a β-blocker (oxprenolol), and selective, left cardiac denervation were evaluated in patients with a first and anterior myocardial infarction. High (n = 144) and low (n = 869) risk groups were identified. The high-risk group consisted of patients who survived a myocardial infarction complicated by either ventricular fibrillation or ventricular tachycardia. The low-risk group consisted of 869 patients who suffered a myocardial infarction without dysrhythmia. The low-risk group was randomized to placebo or β-blockade with oxprenolol. The high-risk group was randomized to placebo, oxprenolol, or left cardiac sympathetic denervation. Crude death rates for each group were determined and both oxprenolol and left cardiac denervation reduced mortality to a level that was significantly lower than observed in the placebo group (**Table 4**).

Group	Mortality rate (%) (n = 144)	p-Value (difference from Placebo group)
Placebo	21.3	–
Oxprenolol	2.7	0.05*
Left cardiac sympathetic denervation	3.6	0.05*

*Statistical significance.

Table 4. Comparison of high risk, postinfarction group mortality rates in the clinical study of pharmacologic and surgical antiadrenergic interventions [87].

The authors concluded that left cardiac sympathetic denervation could be considered as an alternative for high-risk postinfarct patients for whom β-blockade is contraindicated.

Studies which followed this work were anecdotal in nature but tended to iterate this group's findings. Despite lack of randomization and true controls, one study by Coleman et al. [88] examined videoscopic left cardiac sympathetic denervation for patients with recurrent ventricular fibrillation/malignant ventricular fibrillation.

5.3. Sympathetic denervation in genetic channelopathies

The work of Coleman et al. is unique in that they studied the procedure in patients who did not carry the diagnosis of congenital long QT syndrome (LQTS). Their work was a single center, retrospective examination of 91 patients who had videoscopic LCSD, with special attention to the 27 patients in the group who did have LQTS. The dysrythmogenic syndromes from which these patients did suffer included catecholaminergic polymorphic ventricular tachycardia (CPVT) (n = 13); Jervell and Lange-Nielsen syndrome (n = 5) (congenital profound bilateral sensorineural hearing loss and long QTC usually greater than 500 msec iron-deficiency anemia, and elevated levels of gastrin); idiopathic ventricular fibrillation ($n = 4$); left ventricular noncompaction ($n = 2$); hypertrophic cardiomyopathy ($n = 1$); ischemic cardiomyopathy ($n = 1$); and dysrythmogenic right ventricular cardiomyopathy ($n = 1$). Five patients had LCSD because of β-blockade intolerance. The authors concluded that LCSD may represent an antiarrhythmic intervention which is substrate independent for patients with life-threatening ventricular dysrhythmias from causes other than long QT syndrome (**Table 5**) [88].

Syndrome	Total	Post LCSD dysrhythmic event rate
Catecholaminergic polymorphic ventricular tachycardia	13	1/13
Lange-Nielsen syndrome	5	1/5
Idiopathic ventricular fibrillation	4	1/4
Left ventricular non-compaction	2	0/1
Hypertrophic cardiomyopathy	1	1/1
Ischemic cardiomyopathy	1	0/1
Arrythmogenic right ventricular cardiomyopathy	1	0/1

Table 5. Results of LCSD intervention in patients with life-threatening ventricular dysrhythmias from causes other than long Q-T syndrome are shown in this table.

In a small study performed by Nademanee et al. in 2000, 49 patients who had electrical storm associated with a recent (mean 11 ± 10 days) myocardial infarction were divided into two groups in order to study the efficacy of "sympathetic blockade" versus antiarrhythmic agents as recommended by the Advanced Cardiac Life Support guidelines. It should be noted that in this study in the "sympathetic blockade" group, six of the 27 (22%) patients received stellate ganglion block, with seven (26%) receiving esmolol and 14 (52%) receiving propranolol. In the second, ACLS group patients received lidocaine (1 mg/kg IV bolus) followed by continuous infusion of lidocaine (1–4 mg/min). Procainamide boluses of 100 mg were administered, if sinus rhythm was not obtained, up to a total dose of 500–1000 mg. This was followed by a continuous infusion of 2–4 mg/min. Procainamide was used in 16 patients (72%). Bretylium tosylate was given in 18 patients (82%) and administered in 5 mg/kg intravenous boluses and repeated every 5 min up to a maximum dose of 25 mg/kg if the VF recurred. All patients in the group received lidocaine and 12 patients (~55%) received all three drugs at various points in the therapy. In the first week following the event 24 patients died. There were 18 deaths in the ACLS group (82%) and six deaths in the sympathetic blockade group (22%). All deaths in the ACLS group were due to refractory VF. Among the six deaths in the sympathetic blockade group, three were from refractory VF, two were from electro mechanical dissociation and one was due to anoxic encephalopathy leading to asystole. The relative risk of dying in the ACLS group was 3.68 compared to the sympathetic blockade. At 1 year the reported survival rate for the ACLS group 2/22 (9%) as opposed to 20/29 (74%) for the sympathetic blockade group. This study, the authors admit, was limited by the fact that patients could not be randomized to treatment arms because of the emergent nature of electrical storm. Therefore, the initial implementation in both groups of the accepted ACLS protocol occurred regardless of ultimate treatment direction. It should be noted, however, that both groups did demonstrate VF that persisted despite the ACLS and the authors correctly state that because of this there was no apparent predilection toward less refractory or more treatable VF in the sympathetic blockade. One significant omission in this study from our perspective is the lack of further survival analysis in the patients receiving left cardiac sympathetic denervation. These data could impact that rationale for use of LCSD as a standalone intervention. In their discussion, the authors reemphasize the role of increased sympathetic tone in patients with myocardial ischemia and cite animal as well as human studies showing that class I (sodium channel blocking) drugs such as lidocaine and procainamide can increase the risk of asystole and increase the QT interval, respectively [89, 90]. In addition, the authors assert and also correctly cite the fact that class I drugs exert negative inotropic effects and worsen cardiac function, leading to more heart failure, more episodes of ventricular fibrillation in patients who have left ventricular dysfunction, and mild congestive heart failure [91, 92]. The authors propose in conclusion that all patients with ES should be given β-blockers even if they suffer congestive heart failure, left ventricular dysfunction or dysrhythmias that cause hemodynamic compromise.

6. Neural blockade and management of ventricular dysrhythmias

6.1. Technique of stellate ganglion blockade for management of ventricular dysrhythmias

Currently, the stellate ganglion block is typically performed using ultrasound guidance. In the not too distant past, before the advent of ultrasound-guided nerve blocks, the procedure was performed "blind," i.e., using anatomic landmarks. While current practice still relies on anatomic landmarks to acquire the bearings for the block, ultrasound imaging is essential to obtain definitive confirmation that target structures have been visualized and accessed appropriately; and that structures that must be avoided (vascular, respiratory, esophageal, endocrine, etc.) are successfully identified. The linear ultrasound transducer provides the most manageable access to this region.

With the patient in the supine position the lateral neck and the base of the neck are sterilely prepped and draped. The carotid artery is digitally retracted laterally and the ultrasound transducer is positioned close to the longus colli muscle. The transducer is then gently pressed between the carotid artery and trachea at the level of the cricothyroid membrane. This corresponds to the level of the transverse process of the sixth cervical vertebra or Chassaignac's tubercle (**Figure 1**).

An inplane approach (block needle and ultrasound transducer long axes in the same orientation) is used. If a continuous/catheter technique is to be used, an 18 gauge Tuohy is inserted paratracheally toward the middle of the longus colli muscle. The needle insertion endpoint is the ultrasound image demonstrating the tip of needle penetrating the prevertebral fascia in the longus colli (**Figure 2**).

http://dx.doi.org/10.5772/66517

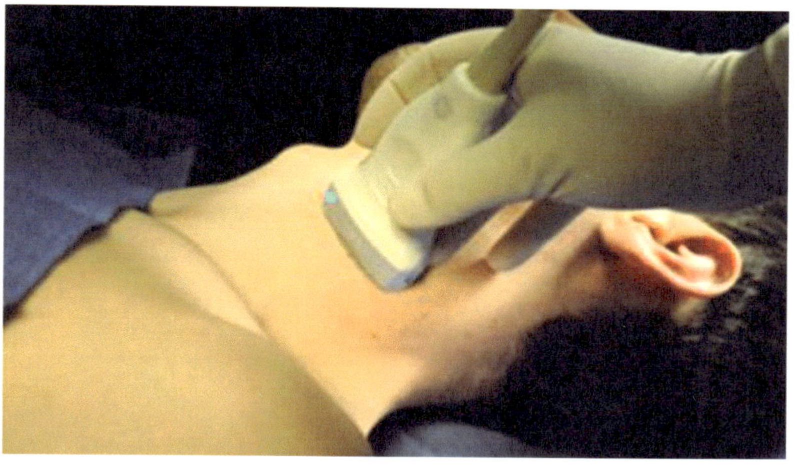

Figure 1. Placement of ultrasound transducer for ultrasound-guided left stellate ganglion block. Courtesy of the New York Society of Regional Anesthesiology (NYSORA).

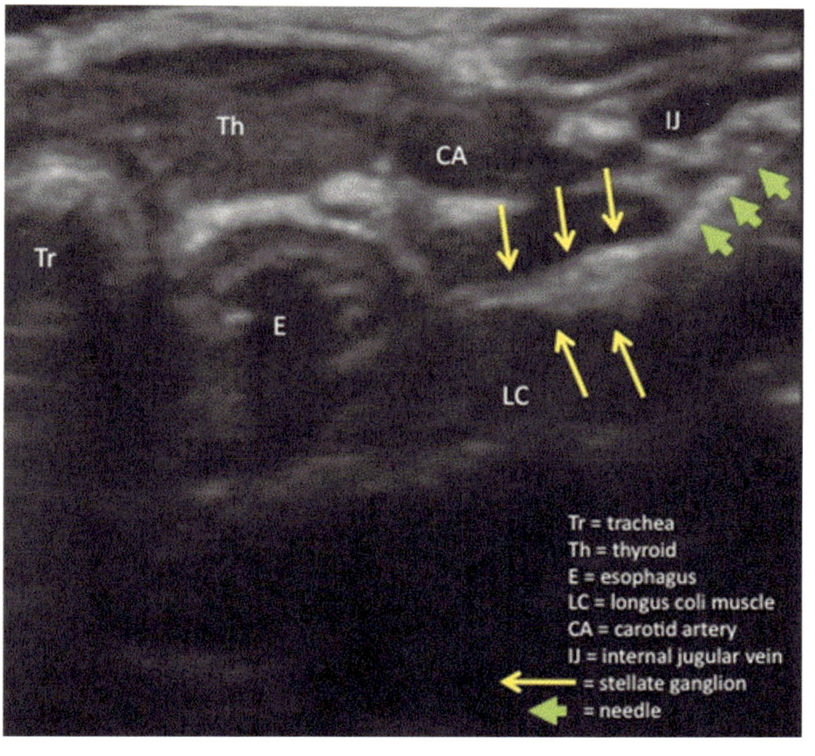

Figure 2. Ultrasound of left stellate ganglion (indicated by long yellow arrows) and related anatomy are shown. Note proximity to the carotid artery (CA) and the internal jugular (IJ) vein. The short green arrows indicate the block needle. Courtesy of the New York Society of Regional Anesthesiology (NYSORA).

Following attainment of the prevertebral fascia of the longus colli muscle, negative aspiration for blood and cerebrospinal fluid must be demonstrated. Local anesthetic is injected and its spread is visualized in real time. Under sterile conditions, a 20 gauge polyethylene catheter is inserted through the Tuohy needle to the left stellate ganglion within the prevertebral fascial layer. An intervascular approach between the left carotid artery and the left internal jugular vein may be used if dictated by anatomical restrictions (**Figure 3**). A continuous infusion of 1 mL per hour of 1% preservative free lidocaine may be initiated [93].

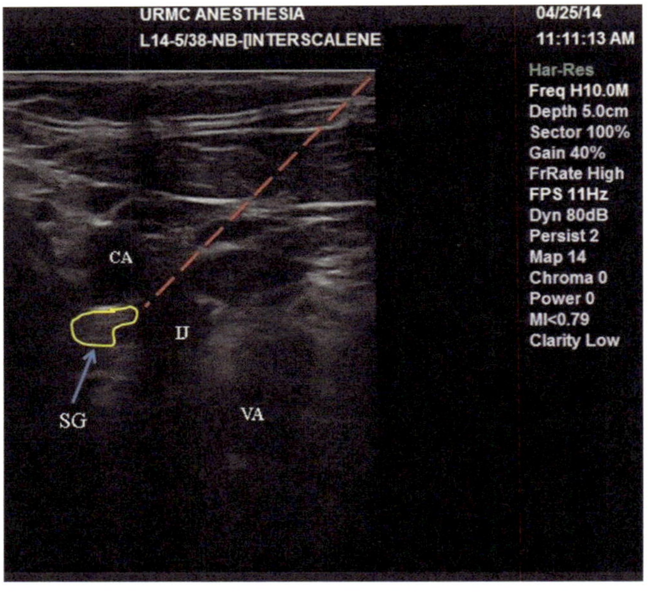

Figure 3. Ultrasound of left stellate ganglion (SG) block using the intervascular approach between carotid area (CA) and internal jugular (IJ) vein is shown. VA is vertebral artery; dashed red line is course of 18 gauge Tuohy needle and subsequent 20 gauge polyethylene catheter [93].

6.2. LCSD for ventricular dysrhythmias: review of case reports in the literature

In his thorough review of the evaluation and management of electrical storm, Effing et al. mentioned left stellate ganglion blockade as a means of suppressing electrical storms that were refracting to multiple antiarrhythmic agents and B-blockade. The review, however, does not mention the anecdotal reports of successful stellate ganglion blockade in VT/VF refractory which is refractory to countershock administered by AICD. At the time of this writing there are five case reports or case series in the recent literature, which address successful use of LCSD accomplished via somewhat different methods to treatment recurrent VT and electrical storm. This section addresses each of these reports in chronologic order and compares the specific clinical settings in which they were used.

In 2009, Collura et al. performed an electronic medical record review of 20 patients at their institution who received LCSD for the treatment of two cardiac channelopathies: long QT syndrome and catecholaminergic polymorphic ventricular tachycardia (CPVT). Their study population consisted of 20 patients with an age range of 2 months to 42 years; with a gender component of 8 females and 12 males. Eighteen of the patients received the VATS procedure and two had a traditional or "open" approach for the LCSD. They reported no intraoperative ectopy, no uncontrolled hemorrhage, and no VATS case requiring conversion to an open approach nor any other perioperative complication in their short term follow-up period (mean 16.6 ± 9.5 months). They found a "marked" reduction in cardiac events in patients (n = 11) who received LCSD as secondary prevention [94].

Mahajan et al. 2005 took a different approach to accomplishing LCSD. In their case report, they describe thoracic epidural anesthesia (TEA) for electrical storm [95]. Their decision to attempt control with TEA was based on extrapolation from the work of Blomberg et al. who found significant symptomatic improvement in patients suffering from intractable angina, in addition to finding attenuation of stress induced myocardial ischemia [96]. Their attempt was also bolstered by the editorial remarks of Staats and Panchal [97] which supported the use of this technique in the coronary care unit for patients with severe angina [97]. In their report, Mahajan et al. describe a 75-year-old man with a history of ischemic cardiomyopathy (LVEF = 20%); an AICD (with 86 shocks and 42 antitachycardia pacing attempts over a 48-h period); and a history of two separate coronary artery bypass grafting procedures 15 years apart. The patient was being treated with maximal antiarrhythmic therapy (mexilitene, amiodarone, nitroglycerine, and esmolol) and deemed ineligible for further coronary revascularization. The patient's AICD battery was depleted and general endotracheal anesthesia was required for radiofrequency ablation and the AICD battery change. The patient continued to have VF/VT despite increasing doses of anesthetics and antidysrhythmics. The patient received an "emergent" thoracic epidural catheter placement in the hope of controlling the dysrhythmias and an infusion was begun. They report that during the time of the epidural infusion only one episode of VF occurred.

Loyalka et al. [98] discuss a 58-year-old male with a history of a complete Q-wave anterior myocardial infarction who developed unstable ventricular dysrhythmias treated with repeated external countershocks. The patient's condition then deteriorated to pulseless ventricular dysrhythmias which required a series of direct current shocks and amiodarone for stabilization. The patient underwent an urgent implantation of a percutaneous ventricular assist device (Tandem Heart) which accomplished left atrial-femoral artery bypass. The dysrhythmias were reported to have persisted at which point a left stellate ganglion block was performed with 0.25% bupivacaine. After the block the patent required a single defibrillation of 200 J and had no further sustained dysrhythmias. Following the procedure, they reported frequent premature ventricular contractions and short 3–5 beat of nonsustained ventricular tachycardia. The patient developed an ectopic atrial tachycardia which was mapped and ablated. He received a dual chamber AICD. The authors correctly note that this is currently the only case found in the literature of such a description to have been successfully treated with left atrial femoral support and left stellate ganglion block [98].

In 2014, Malik et al. reported the successful treatment of a 70-year-old man who suffered from ischemic cardiomyopathy and had an AICD. The patient had developed intractable VT which was resistant to amiodarone, lidocaine, and multiple unsuccessful radiofrequency catheter ablation attempts of the ectopic foci. The patient continued to have up to 18 AICD shockable events per day. At 2.5 h, following a stellate ganglion block the ventricular tachycardia reverted to a normal sinus rhythm which persisted for at least 1 month which is the latest reported follow-up in the case study [99].

Finally, in 2015 this author (Smith et al.) published a report of a 65-year-old male with a diagnosis of electric storm and a history of nonischemic cardiomyopathy, prostate cancer, and a previously placed left ventricular assist device. The patient received a continuous left stellate ganglion block which was continued for 7 days. Based upon the result of this block, a surgical (open technique) left cardiac sympathetic denervation was performed. It was important for us in this case to establish a continuous left sympathetic blockade infusion for 6 days in order minimize the likelihood that we were simply observing a period of spontaneous ectopic quiescence [93]. No definitive studies have addressed specifically the optimal time for blockade before definitive treatment is employed. At our institution, we also used 1 week by convention to allow for reversal of the patients' coumadin therapy with bridging using a heparin infusion during this period. At the same time, in each of our cases, there was a marked reduction in the number of episodes of daily shockable events (DSEs). Statistical analysis of the number of individuals treated by this technique at our institution remains too small for rigorous statistical analysis. We did however look at the mean number of DSE both prior to and following each intervention over a 6 day week or a 144 h period considered as 144 sample times. In our observations, we found no noticeable difference in the number of DSE's between the postblock and the postsurgical interventions. We found that differences between DSE preintervention and postblock did exist and examined these on an intrapatient basis. For differences between preintervention and postintervention, we used a repeat measures *t*-test and found a preintervention DSE value (5.5 ± 4.04) postblock DSE (0.38 ± 4.04). We looked at the two patients in whom we proceeded to permanent blockade and found intrapatient differences in DSE value. We used the same mean overall DSE in the eight total patients and defined that as our "population" (5.5 ± 4.04). This was done despite the fact that the mean DSE in the two patients who preceded to permanent denervation techniques was higher than in the "population." Our intention here was to more critically compare the differences pre and postintervention and to reduce bias as well. We found intrapatient differences at the $p \leq 0.004$ and $p \leq 0.0048$ levels, respectively. Currently, we use these determinations applied to intrapatient results to direct our care on a case by case basis. **Table 6** presents the summary of case studies in the literature which employed LCSD for ventricular tachydysrhythmias.

Study, (year)	Type of work	N	Population,(patient)	Clinical setting	Technique	Outcome	Comment
Mahajan et al. [95]	Case report	1	75-year-old man	ES, LVEF; antidysrhythmic therapy failure	Thoracic epidural	Cessation of sustained VT	Proceeded to get VAD (left atrial—femoral bypass)
Collura et al. [94]	Retrospective electronic chart analysis	20	2-months old to 42-years old (8 female, 20 male)	LQTS and CPVT	Surgical ganglionectomy; 18 VATS and two open	No perioperative ectopy; no hemorrhage; no VATS – open conversion determined safety of procedure*	Marked reduction in cardiac events in post getting LCSD as secondary prevention
Loyalka et al. [98]	Case report	1	58-year-old man	Anterior MI; unstable VT; repeated external countershocks; amiodarone	Stellate ganglion block (single)	1 Post-procedure defibrillation. No further events.	Ablation of developed ectopic atrial tachycardic focus; AICD placement
Malik et al. [99]	Case report	1	70-year-old man	Ischemic cardiomyopathy, AICD, intractable VT; failed RF ablation; ES	Stellate ganglion block (single)	VT reverted to NSR 2.5 h after block. Lasted through one month follow-up period	
Smith et al. [93]	Case report	1	65-year-old-man	ES, AICD, LVAD	Continuous stellate ganglion block	Open surgical ganglionectomy performed at day 7 of continuous block based on results	

Table 6. Summary of the case study literature on stellate ganglion blockade for ventricular tachydysrhythmia.

7. Anticoagulation considerations for neural blockade for management of ventricular dysrhythmias

The incidence of hemorrhagic complications associated with neuraxial blockade is not known but has been cited as 1 in 150,000 epidurals and 1 in 220,000 spinals in the literature. Recent epidemiologic data suggest that in certain populations, the incidence may be higher. Because of the proximity of the stellate ganglion to the neuraxis and the potentially catastrophic consequences of intracervical hemorrhage, we treat this block as if were a neuraxial block and apply the same precautions used in actual neuraxial injections [100]. Underlying abnormalities of the spinal cord, preexisting coagulopathy, increasing age, difficulty placing needle, and indwelling neuraxial catheter in the setting of sustained anticoagulation are risk factors for clinically significant bleeding associated with neuraxial and certain regional blockade techniques [101]. These present challenges for clinicians performing regional anesthesia in such patients. Due to the safety concerns of bleeding risk, several agencies including American Society of Regional Anesthesia (ASRA), American College of Chest Physicians (ACCP), and European Society of Regional Anesthesia (ESRA) have provided guidelines and recommendations to reduce patient morbidity/mortality during regional anesthesia. For patients taking anticoagulants, these guidelines and recommendations for practicing regional anesthesia are based on available evidence from epidemiologic data with the goals of making hospital-based medical practice standard, optimizing patient outcomes, and ensuring quality patient care [102]. Variation from these recommendations may be acceptable since no specific clinical outcome can be guaranteed from the suggested guidelines. Patient factors as mentioned earlier, clinician expertise and choice of materials/medications can influence clinical outcome and experience.

There are no current laboratory models and cervical hematomas are rare which makes constructing prospective-randomized studies a challenge. These practice guidelines or recommendations are therefore a summary of evidence-based reviews and the collective experience of recognized experts in regional anesthesia and anticoagulation [102]. To this end, the decision to perform stellate ganglion blockade (either via single injection or via continuous infusion catheter), and the timing of catheter removal in a patient receiving antithrombotic therapy should be made on an individual basis, taking into account the risk of cervical hematoma with the benefits of regional anesthesia for a specific patient. Published guidelines and recommendations should be used to mitigate confusion.

Understanding pharmacokinetics and pharmacodynamics of anticoagulation therapy, timing of administration and determining the appropriate time to conduct a safe procedure is essential to performing regional anesthesia in an anticoagulated patient [103]. Alternative anesthetic and analgesic techniques should be considered in patients with an unacceptable risk. However, some of these recommendations should be applied when performing regional anesthesia in every patient on anticoagulation. Coagulation status should be optimized at the time of sympathetic neural needle/catheter placement, and the level of anticoagulation must be carefully monitored during the period of perineural catheterization [102]. Indwelling catheters should not be removed in the setting of therapeutic anticoagulation as removal seems to significantly increase the risk of hematoma. Identification of risk factors and establishment of guidelines will not completely eliminate complication of regional anesthesia in an anticoagulated patient. Vigilance in monitoring is critical to allow early evaluation of neurologic dysfunction and prompt intervention. Protocols must be in place for urgent magnetic resonance imaging and hematoma evacuation if there is a change in neurologic status. We must focus not only on the prevention of intracervical or perineural hematoma but also on rapid diagnosis and treatment to optimize patient outcome.

8. Ventricular dysrhythmias and AICD-discharge-related anxiety syndromes

In some patients, the persistence of ventricular dysrhythmias and subsequent AICD discharges can have distressing effects. This becomes a vicious cycle in which the shock itself and anticipation of the pain and discomfort associated with the shock can cause significant anxiety, increase the level of hormones associated with stress, and thus, potentially increase the incidence of adrenergic-susceptible ventricle tachyarrhythmias. The data on this phenomenon are not absolutely consistent. At least one study reports the absence of impact on emotional distress. In 2003, Ladwig et al. described 37 patients with chronic atrial fibrillation, mean age 61.9 with a gender breakdown of 29 men and 8 women. They assessed pain perceptions of low energy test shocks (60 V, O.1 J) immediately following the discharge. The group also collected data from the patients regarding treatment anxiety, depression, and somatization. Forty one percent of patients (n = 15) perceived the shocks as hypalgesic, 10 patients (27%) perceived it as normalgesic and 12 patients (32%) perceived it as hyperalgesic. They also noted that the pain threshold was significantly lower ($p \leq 0.029$) in patients in which AF was accidentally diagnosed and an inappropriate discharge was delivered. They state that the hyperalgesic pain threshold was not associated with anxiety depression, or the patient's tendency to amplify benign bodily sensations [104]. It should be noted that while this study aims to examine the impact of countershocks on patient emotional status, and pain perception, it may be nonrepresentative in at least two ways. First, the dysrhythmias examined are atrial and it is unclear whether the patient experience can be extrapolated to the ventricular dysrhythmia setting. Second, the experimental protocol in this work used a low-energy test shock of 60 V, 0.1 J. The mean energy delivered for ventricular defibrillation is reported to be 10 J, with maximum shock energies ranging between 25 and 42 J with many monomorphic tachycardias terminable with shocks of 1 J or less [105]. The authors also state that low-energy cardioversion should always be backed up by successive high-energy shocks, since ventricular dysrhythmias can accelerate after low-energy shocks [106]. Thus, even when low-energy cardioversion is used in the ventricular dysrhythmia setting it is frequently still 10-fold greater than that reported in the Ledwig study on atrial dysrhythmias.

The remainders of the studies that examine psychological effects of AICD discharge do report some negative impact on emotional well-being and quality of life (QoL). These studies emphasize various aspects of life that are worth mentioning since the control of the total number of AICD discharges as well as the effective management of electrical storm is the goal of LCSD.

The advent of advanced cardiac support interventions will undoubtedly lead to more patients surviving recurrent VT. In this regard, LCSD should be considered more frequently since the number of patients living with this diagnosis will increase and lead to an overall increase in the number of individuals suffering a decrease in QoL. These patients will likely enter the palliative care setting. We will look at some of these studies chronologically with the ultimate goal of understanding how LCSD may possibly impact those Q0L components.

One of the earliest descriptions of the psychiatric syndromes identified in patients with AICD was given by Fricchione et al. in 1989 and included anxiety, psychological dependence, abuse, and withdrawal [107]. Later Hamner and his group examined three cases involving patients with AICD. He reported that all the patients met the criteria for PTSD based on DSM-IV criteria, i.e., stressor, intrusive recollection, avoidance/numbing, hyper-arousal, duration (greater than one month), and functional significance (causes impairment in important areas of functioning [108]. In the first patient, Hammer describes the resolution of the PTSD, came in the form of the addition of fluoxetine to his established regimen which included amitriptyline and lorazepam. This was followed by cardiac transplantation and subsequent removal of his AICD. The remaining two patients in the case study were treated with either a dual reuptake inhibitor of serotonin and norepinephrine (duloxetine), or a selective serotonin reuptake inhibitor (paroxetine) antidepressant, and psychotherapy in combination with preestablished anxiolytics and tricyclic antidepressants. The group emphasized the important potential for the development of PTSD secondary to AICDs. They correctly state that the effectiveness of psychotherapy and/or psychopharmacology in treating AICD related PTSD has not been systematically investigated [108].

In a 1999 literature review, Sears et al. concluded that 13–38% of AICD recipients experienced diagnosable levels of anxiety with rates of clinical depression that were comparable to other cardiac patient populations. They reported AICD-related concerns, e.g., fear of shock, fear of device malfunction, fear of death, and fear of embarrassment. They concluded that young recipients and those with high discharge rates may experience the most adjustment difficulties [109].

Two papers published in 2002 turned focus onto QoL issues by distinct definition. In that year, Sears et al. [110] compared QoL studies that examined antidysrhythmic therapy with AICD. They noted that the primary focus of these studies was upon mortality rather than AICD-specific and antiarrhythmic-specific measures that may be more sensitive to psychological outcomes. They stated that the existing work suggested that the ICD achieved comparable if not better QoL than alternative treatments, but stated that future measurements and interventions should focus on patient acceptance of the device. The group also recommended that routine integration of psychosocial needs considerations should be added to the clinical care of patients with AICD. Also, in 2002, Schron et al. provided three self-administered instruments to measure generic and disease specific QoL in the antiarrhthmics versus implantable defibrillators (AVIDs) trial participants. They reported that overall AICD and antiarrhythmic drugs (AAD) were associated with similar alterations in QoL with the development of sporadic shocks and adverse symptoms associated with reduced physical functioning and mental well-being and increased concerns among ICD recipients; and reduced physical functioning and increased concerns among AAD recipients [111].

In another study that focused on the psycho social impact of AICD on spouses, Sowell et al. in 2007 examined patients and their spouses (n = 62) who completed separate individual assessment batteries regarding demographics, death anxiety, shock anxiety, general anxiety, and marital adjustment at a single time point during outpatient cardiology visits. Their results revealed similar general anxiety and marital adjustment among participants with spouses actually reporting greater shock anxiety than did the patients themselves ($p = 0.045$). The study also revealed that female ICD patients reported more anxiety related to death and shock and received more shocks given identical degrees of clinical severity ($p = 0.02$) [112].

In what may the most definitive study to date, Mark et al. in a randomized trial compared AICD therapy or amiodarone with state of the art medical therapy alone, found that psychological well-being in the AICD group, as compared with medical therapy alone was significantly improved at 3 months ($p = 0.01$) at 12 months ($p = 0.003$); but not at 30 months. It should be emphasized that this study not only compared to AICD and medical therapy but also examined changes in scores on the medical outcomes study 36 item short form (SF-36) scale for patients who had received an ICD shock which they calculated as the difference between the most recent overall QoL category score that existed prior to the shock and that which the patient noted immediately following a shock. In each of the five categories (general health perceptions, physical function, emotional function, social function, and self-rated health) there were statistically significant decrements in QoL [113].

9. Summary

The summary of the progression from diagnosis to treatment with LCSD described in this chapter is found below.

The use of neural blockade has thus far been applied as a last resort [88] in the treatment of malignant ventricular tachyarrhythmias in the setting of heart failure. This chapter has examined the progression of therapeutic intervention from least invasive (pharmacologic only) to the most invasive techniques and interventions. Whether or not this is the optimal organizational approach to these maladies is difficult to discern. Given the acuity and the potential severity of the ventricular tachyarrhythmias, it is extraordinarily difficult to construct true randomized, controlled trials in human subjects to specifically answer these questions and potentially optimize the progression from one treatment modality to the next. In the future, modifications in all aspects of care for these patients will no doubt be addressed particularly with regard to how specific neural blockade of the left cardiac sympathetic innervation can be implemented in a more timely and patient-convenient fashion with the goal of overall improvement in clinical outcomes of survival as well as in quality of life.

Pharmacologic Intervention

- **β- Blockade (Associated with Decreased Mortality)**
- **Amiodarone**
  - Used for Acute Hemodynamic Unstable Ventricular
  - No Demographic Improvement in Survival

Implantable Devices ± Pharmacologic Intervention

- **AICD**: Single Shock Only- Reduces Mortality by 23%
  - At 5 years Overall Mortality is reduced by 7%
- **CRT- P**: indicated for Systolic Heart Failure with QRS ≥ 120 msec.
- **CRT- D**: Indicated for Ischemic Cardiomyopathy
  - 30% risk of SCD Reduction Compared to **CRT-P**

Ablative Techniques

- **Indication**
  - Unifocal Ventricular Ectopic Beats Arising from the RVOT
  - Treatment of Monomorphism Yields Greatest Result
  - More Difficult in the Setting of Structural Heart Disease Because of Larger Size of the Re-Entrant Circuit

Neural Blockade to Interrupt Adrenergic Innervation

- **Stellate Ganglion Blockade**
  - Most Common
  - Single Injection Technique
  - Continuous SGB Technique if Plan to Proceed to "Permanent" Interruption
- **Continuous Thoracic Epidural Technique**
  - Has Been Effective in one Reported case
- **Surgical Ganglionectomy**
  - May be used following trial of Pharmacological Ganglionic Blockade

Author details

Daryl I. Smith* and Albert O. Duah

*Address all correspondence to: daryl_smith@urmc.rochester.edu

Acute Pain Service, Department of Anesthesiology, University of Rochester, School of Medicine and Dentistry, University of Rochester Medical Center, Rochester, New York, USA

References

[1] Joseph, S.M., et al., Acute decompensated heart failure: contemporary medical management. Tex Heart Inst J, 2009. **36**(6): pp. 510–20.

[2] Chakko, C.S. and M. Gheorghiade, Ventricular arrhythmias in severe heart failure: incidence, significance, and effectiveness of antiarrhythmic therapy. Am Heart J, 1985. **109**(3 Pt 1): pp. 497–504.

[3] Poole-Wilson, P.A., et al., Mode of death in heart failure: findings from the ATLAS trial. Heart, 2003. **89**(1): pp. 42–8.

[4] Kennedy, H.L., et al., Long-term follow-up of asymptomatic healthy subjects with frequent and complex ventricular ectopy. N Engl J Med, 1985. **312**(4): pp. 193–7.

[5] Lerma, C., et al., Patterns of ectopy leading to increased risk of fatal or near-fatal cardiac arrhythmia in patients with depressed left ventricular function after an acute myocardial infarction. Europace, 2013. **15**(9): pp. 1304–12.

[6] Doval, H.C., et al., Nonsustained ventricular tachycardia in severe heart failure. Independent marker of increased mortality due to sudden death. GESICA-GEMA Investigators. Circulation, 1996. **94**(12): pp. 3198–203.

[7] Pogwizd, S.M. and P.B. Corr, Mechanisms underlying the development of ventricular fibrillation during early myocardial ischemia. Circ Res, 1990. **66**(3): pp. 672–95.

[8] Calkins, H., et al., Catheter ablation of ventricular tachycardia in patients with structural heart disease using cooled radiofrequency energy: results of a prospective multicenter study. Cooled RF Multi Center Investigators Group. J Am Coll Cardiol, 2000. **35**(7): pp. 1905–14.

[9] Effing, M., M. Razavi, and A. Masumi, The evaluation and management of electrical storm. Tex heart Inst J, 2011. **38**(2): pp. 111–21.

[10] Oppenheimer, S.M., et al., Insular cortex stimulation produces lethal cardiac arrhythmias: a mechanism of sudden death? Brain Res, 1991. **550**(1): pp. 115–21.

[11] Hasan, W., Autonomic cardiac innervation: development and adult plasticity. Organogenesis, 2013. **9**(3): pp. 176–93.

[12] Conlon, K., T. Collins, and C. Kidd, Modulation of vagal actions on heart rate produced by inhibition of nitric oxide synthase in the anaesthetized ferret. Exp Physiol, 1996. **81**(3): pp. 547–50.

[13] Henning, R.J. and D.R. Sawmiller, Vasoactive intestinal peptide: cardiovascular effects. Cardiovasc Res, 2001. **49**(1): pp. 27–37.

[14] Protas, L., J. Qu, and R.B. Robinson, Neuropeptide y: neurotransmitter or trophic factor in the heart? News Physiol Sci, 2003. **18**: pp. 181–5.

[15] Ernsberger, U., The development of postganglionic sympathetic neurons: coordinating neuronal differentiation and diversification. Auton Neurosci, 2001. **94**(1–2): pp. 1–13.

[16] Testut, L. and A. Latarjet, Human Anatomy. Vol. 2. 1961,Salvat: Barcelona, Spain.

[17] Pardini, B.J., D.D. Lund, and P.G. Schmid, Organization of the sympathetic postganglionic innervation of the rat heart. J Auton Nerv Syst, 1989. **28**(3): pp. 193–201.

[18] Pardini, B.J., D.D. Lund, and P.G. Schmid, Innervation patterns of the middle cervical--stellate ganglion complex in the rat. Neurosci Lett, 1990. **117**(3): pp. 300–6.

[19] Waldmann, M., et al., Stochastic behavior of atrial and ventricular intrinsic cardiac neurons. J Appl Physiol (1985), 2006. **101**(2): pp. 413–9.

[20] Thompson, G.W., et al., Functional interdependence of neurons in a single canine intrinsic cardiac ganglionated plexus. J Physiol, 2000. **528**(Pt 3): pp. 561–71.

[21] Randall, D.C., et al., Interactions within the intrinsic cardiac nervous system contribute to chronotropic regulation. Am J Physiol Regul Integr Comp Physiol, 2003. **285**(5): pp. R1066–75.

[22] Olshansky, B., Interrelationships between the autonomic nervous system and atrial fibrillation. Prog Cardiovasc Dis, 2005. **48**(1): pp. 57–78.

[23] Armour, J.A., Intrinsic cardiac neurons involved in cardiac regulation possess alpha 1-, alpha 2-, beta 1- and beta 2-adrenoceptors. Can J Cardiol, 1997. **13**(3): pp. 277–84.

[24] Chen, P.S., et al., Sympathetic nerve sprouting, electrical remodeling and the mechanisms of sudden cardiac death. Cardiovasc Res, 2001. **50**(2): pp. 409–16.

[25] Prichard, B.N., The second Lilly Prize Lecture, University of Newcastle, July 1977. beta-Adrenergic receptor blockade in hypertension, past, present and future. Br J Clin Pharmacol, 1978. **5**(5): pp. 379–99.

[26] Naccarelli, G.V., et al., A decade of clinical trial developments in postmyocardial infarction, congestive heart failure, and sustained ventricular tachyarrhythmia patients: from CAST to AVID and beyond. Cardiac Arrhythmic Suppression Trial. Antiarrhythmic Versus Implantable Defibrillators. J Cardiovasc Electrophysiol, 1998. **9**(8): pp. 864–91.

[27] Baker, J.G., S.J. Hill, and R.J. Summers, Evolution of beta-blockers: from anti-anginal drugs to ligand-directed signalling. Trends Pharmacol Sci, 2011. **32**(4): pp. 227–34.

[28] Prichard, B.N. and P.M. Gillam, Use of propranolol (inderal) in treatment of hypertension. Br Med J, 1964. **2**(5411): pp. 725–7.

[29] Waldo, A.L., et al., Effect of d-sotalol on mortality in patients with left ventricular dysfunction after recent and remote myocardial infarction. The SWORD Investigators. Survival with Oral d-Sotalol. Lancet, 1996. **348**(9019): pp. 7–12.

[30] Schwartz, P.J., M.T. La Rovere, and E. Vanoli, Autonomic nervous system and sudden cardiac death. Experimental basis and clinical observations for post-myocardial infarction risk stratification. Circulation, 1992. **85**(1 Suppl): pp. I77–91.

[31] Echt, D.S., et al., Mortality and morbidity in patients receiving encainide, flecainide, or placebo. The Cardiac Arrhythmia Suppression Trial. N Engl J Med, 1991. **324**(12): pp. 781–8.

[32] Effect of the antiarrhythmic agent moricizine on survival after myocardial infarction. The Cardiac Arrhythmia Suppression Trial II Investigators. N Engl J Med, 1992. **327**(4): pp. 227–33.

[33] Tepper, D., Frontiers in congestive heart failure: effect of metoprolol CR/XL in chronic heart failure: metoprolol CR/XL randomised intervention trial in congestive heart failure (MERIT-HF). Congest Heart Fail, 1999. **5**(4): pp. 184–185.

[34] McMurray, J., et al., Antiarrhythmic effect of carvedilol after acute myocardial infarction: results of the carvedilol post-infarct survival control in left ventricular dysfunction (CAPRICORN) trial. J Am Coll Cardiol, 2005. **45**(4): pp. 525–30.

[35] The Cardiac Insufficiency Bisoprolol Study II (CIBIS-II): a randomised trial. Lancet, 1999. **353**(9146): pp. 9–13.

[36] Bardy, G.H., et al., Amiodarone or an implantable cardioverter-defibrillator for congestive heart failure. N Engl J Med, 2005. **352**(3): pp. 225–37.

[37] Cairns, J.A., et al., Randomised trial of outcome after myocardial infarction in patients with frequent or repetitive ventricular premature depolarisations: CAMIAT. Canadian Amiodarone Myocardial Infarction Arrhythmia Trial Investigators. Lancet, 1997. **349**(9053): pp. 675–82.

[38] Singh, S.N., P.E. Carson, and S.G. Fisher, Nonsustained ventricular tachycardia in severe heart failure. Circulation, 1997. **96**(10): pp. 3794–5.

[39] Singh, S.N., et al., Amiodarone in patients with congestive heart failure and asymptomatic ventricular arrhythmia. Survival trial of antiarrhythmic therapy in congestive heart failure. N Engl J Med, 1995. **333**(2): pp. 77–82.

[40] Kober, L., et al., Effect of dofetilide in patients with recent myocardial infarction and left-ventricular dysfunction: a randomised trial. Lancet, 2000. **356**(9247): pp. 2052–8.

[41] Belhassen, B., et al., Idiopathic recurrent sustained ventricular tachycardia responsive to verapamil: an ECG-electrophysiologic entity. Am Heart J, 1984. **108**(4 Pt 1): pp. 1034–7.

[42] Gill, J.S., et al., Verapamil for the suppression of idiopathic ventricular tachycardia of left bundle branch block-like morphology. Am Heart J, 1993. **126**(5): pp. 1126–33.

[43] Sung, R.J., et al., Effects of verapamil on ventricular tachycardias possibly caused by reentry, automaticity, and triggered activity. J Clin Invest, 1983. **72**(1): pp. 350–60.

[44] Thomas, K.L., et al., Amiodarone use after acute myocardial infarction complicated by heart failure and/or left ventricular dysfunction may be associated with excess mortality. Am Heart J, 2008. **155**(1): pp. 87–93.

[45] Torp-Pedersen, C., et al., The safety of amiodarone in patients with heart failure. J Card Fail, 2007. **13**(5): pp. 340–5.

[46] Bauman, A.L., et al., Dynamic regulation of cAMP synthesis through anchored PKA-adenylyl cyclase V/VI complexes. Mol Cell, 2006. **23**(6): pp. 925–31.

[47] Bos, J.L., Epac: a new cAMP target and new avenues in cAMP research. Nat Rev Mol Cell Biol, 2003. **4**(9): pp. 733–8.

[48] Zaccolo, M. and T. Pozzan, Discrete microdomains with high concentration of cAMP in stimulated rat neonatal cardiac myocytes. Science, 2002. **295**(5560): pp. 1711–5.

[49] Dodge-Kafka, K.L., et al., The protein kinase A anchoring protein mAKAP coordinates two integrated cAMP effector pathways. Nature, 2005. **437**(7058): pp. 574–8.

[50] Metrich, M., et al., Role of the cAMP-binding protein Epac in cardiovascular physiology and pathophysiology. Pflugers Arch, 2010. **459**(4): pp. 535–46.

[51] Morel, E., et al., cAMP-binding protein Epac induces cardiomyocyte hypertrophy. Circ Res, 2005. **97**(12): pp. 1296–304.

[52] Rajagopal, S., K. Rajagopal, and R.J. Lefkowitz, Teaching old receptors new tricks: biasing seven-transmembrane receptors. Nat Rev Drug Discov, 2010. **9**(5): pp. 373–86.

[53] Kamp, T.J. and J.W. Hell, Regulation of cardiac L-type calcium channels by protein kinase A and protein kinase C. Circ Res, 2000. **87**(12): pp. 1095–102.

[54] Thomas, G.D., Neural control of the circulation. Adv Physiol Educ, 2011. **35**(1): pp. 28–32.

[55] Lipscombe, D., L-type calcium channels: highs and new lows. Circ Res, 2002. **90**(9): pp. 933–5.

[56] Buxton, A.E., et al., A randomized study of the prevention of sudden death in patients with coronary artery disease. Multicenter unsustained tachycardia trial investigators. N Engl J Med, 1999. **341**(25): pp. 1882–90.

[57] Tang, A.S., et al., Cardiac-resynchronization therapy for mild-to-moderate heart failure. N Engl J Med, 2010. **363**(25): pp. 2385–95.

[58] Epstein, A.E., et al., ACC/AHA/HRS 2008 guidelines for device-based therapy of cardiac rhythm abnormalities: a report of the American College of Cardiology/American Heart Association Task Force on Practice Guidelines (Writing Committee to Revise the ACC/AHA/NASPE 2002 Guideline Update for Implantation of Cardiac Pacemakers and Antiarrhythmia Devices): developed in collaboration with the American Association for Thoracic Surgery and Society of Thoracic Surgeons. Circulation, 2008. **117**(21): pp. e350–408.

[59] Kusumoto, F.M., et al., HRS/ACC/AHA expert consensus statement on the use of implantable cardioverter-defibrillator therapy in patients who are not included or not well represented in clinical trials. Circulation, 2014. **130**(1): pp. 94–125.

[60] Tracy, C.M., et al., 2012 ACCF/AHA/HRS focused update of the 2008 guidelines for device-based therapy of cardiac rhythm abnormalities: a report of the American College of Cardiology Foundation/American Heart Association Task Force on Practice Guidelines and the Heart Rhythm Society. [corrected]. Circulation, 2012. **126**(14): pp. 1784–800.

[61] Yancy, C.W., et al., 2013 ACCF/AHA guideline for the management of heart failure: executive summary: a report of the American College of Cardiology Foundation/American Heart Association Task Force on practice guidelines. Circulation, 2013. **128**(16): pp. 1810–52.

[62] Zipes, D.P., et al., ACC/AHA/ESC 2006 guidelines for management of patients with ventricular arrhythmias and the prevention of sudden cardiac death: a report of the American College of Cardiology/American Heart Association Task Force and the European Society of Cardiology Committee for Practice Guidelines (writing committee to develop guidelines for management of patients with ventricular arrhythmias and the prevention of sudden cardiac death): developed in collaboration with the European Heart Rhythm Association and the Heart Rhythm Society. Circulation, 2006. **114**(10): pp. e385–484.

[63] Schoeller, R., et al., First- or second-degree atrioventricular block as a risk factor in idiopathic dilated cardiomyopathy. Am J Cardiol, 1993. **71**(8): pp. 720–6.

[64] Cazeau, S., et al., Four chamber pacing in dilated cardiomyopathy. Pacing Clin Electrophysiol, 1994. **17**(11 Pt 2): pp. 1974–9.

[65] Zweier, J.L., C.A. Chen, and M.A. Talukder, Cardiac resynchronization therapy and reverse molecular remodeling: importance of mitochondrial redox signaling. Circ Res, 2011. **109**(7): pp. 716–9.

[66] Scheffer, M. and B.M. van Gelder, Implantation Techniques of Leads for Left Ventricular Pacing in Cardiac Resynchronization Therapy and Electrocardiographic Consequences of the Stimulation Site in Advances in Electrocardiograms-Methods and Analysis, R. Mills, (ed), Editor. 2012, InTech: Rijeka, Croatia.

[67] Betts, T.R., et al., Development of a technique for left ventricular endocardial pacing via puncture of the interventricular septum. Circ Arrhythm Electrophysiol, 2014. **7**(1): pp. 17–22.

[68] Khan, F.Z., et al., Left ventricular lead placement in cardiac resynchronization therapy: where and how? Europace, 2009. **11**(5): pp. 554–61.

[69] Jiang, M., B. He, and Q. Zhang, Comparison of CRT and CRT-D in heart failure: systematic review of controlled trials. Int J Cardiol, 2012. **158**(1): pp. 39–45.

[70] Gold, M.R., et al., Implantable defibrillators improve survival in patients with mildly symptomatic heart failure receiving cardiac resynchronization therapy: analysis of the long-term follow-up of remodeling in systolic left ventricular dysfunction (REVERSE). Circ Arrhythm Electrophysiol, 2013. **6**(6): pp. 1163–8.

[71] Bristow, M.R., et al., Cardiac-resynchronization therapy with or without an implantable defibrillator in advanced chronic heart failure. N Engl J Med, 2004. **350**(21): pp. 2140–50.

[72] Kutyifa, V., et al., Effect of cardiac resynchronization therapy with implantable cardioverter defibrillator versus cardiac resynchronization therapy with pacemaker on mortality in heart failure patients: results of a high-volume, single-centre experience. Eur J Heart Fail, 2014. **16**(12): pp. 1323–30.

[73] Siontis, K., et al., Radiofrequency ablation versus antiarrhythmic drug therapy for atrial fibrillation: meta-analysis of quality of life, morbidity, and mortality. JACC Clin Electrophysiol, 2016. **2**(2): pp. 170–180.

[74] Morillo, C.A., et al., Radiofrequency ablation vs antiarrhythmic drugs as first-line treatment of paroxysmal atrial fibrillation (RAAFT-2): a randomized trial. JAMA, 2014. **311**(7): pp. 692–700.

[75] Ng, G.A., Treating patients with ventricular ectopic beats. Heart, 2006. **92**(11): pp. 1707–12.

[76] Kottkamp, H., et al., Radiofrequency catheter ablation of sustained ventricular tachycardia in idiopathic dilated cardiomyopathy. Circulation, 1995. **92**(5): pp. 1159–68.

[77] Israel, C.W. and S.S. Barold, Electrical storm in patients with an implanted defibrillator: a matter of definition. Ann Noninvasive Electrocardiol, 2007. **12**(4): pp. 375–82.

[78] Francois-Frank, C.A., Signification physiologique de la resection du sympathetique dans la malade de basedow, l'epilepsie, l'idiotic et la glaucoma bull. Acad Med Paris, 1899. **41**: pp. 565–594.

[79] Jonnesco, T., Traitement chirurgical l'angine de poitrine par le resection du sympathetique cervico-thoracique. Presse Med, 1921. **20**: pp. 221–230.

[80] Schwartz, P.J., Cardiac sympathetic denervation to prevent life-threatening arrhythmias. Nat Rev Cardiol, 2014. **11**(6): pp. 346–53.

[81] Swetlow, G.I., Angina pectoris paravertebral alcohol block for the relief of pain. The American J Surg, 1930. **9**(1): pp. 88–97.

[82] Estes, E.H., Jr. and H.L. Izlar, Jr., Recurrent ventricular tachycardia. A case successfully treated by bilateral cardiac sympathectomy. Am J Med, 1961. **31**: pp. 493–7.

[83] Zipes, D.P., et al., Treatment of ventricular arrhythmia by permanent atrial pacemaker and cardiac sympathectomy. Ann Intern Med, 1968. **68**(3): pp. 591–7.

[84] Fowlis, R.A., et al., Experimental coronary artery ligation in conscious dogs six months after bilateral cardiac sympathectomy. Am Heart J, 1974. **88**(6): pp. 748–57.

[85] Schwartz, P.J. and H.L. Stone, Left stellectomy in the prevention of ventricular fibrillation caused by acute myocardial ischemia in conscious dogs with anterior myocardial infarction. Circulation, 1980. **62**(6): pp. 1256–65.

[86] Moss, A.J. and J. McDonald, Unilateral cervicothoracic sympathetic ganglionectomy for the treatment of long QT interval syndrome. N Engl J Med, 1971. **285**(16): pp. 903–4.

[87] Schwartz, P.J., et al., Prevention of sudden cardiac death after a first myocardial infarction by pharmacologic or surgical antiadrenergic interventions. J Cardiovasc Electrophysiol, 1992. **3**: pp. 2–16.

[88] Coleman, M.A., et al., Videoscopic left cardiac sympathetic denervation for patients with recurrent ventricular fibrillation/malignant ventricular arrhythmia syndromes besides congenital long-QT syndrome. Circ Arrhythm Electrophysiol, 2012. **5**(4): pp. 782–8.

[89] Nattel, S., D.H. Pedersen, and D.P. Zipes, Alterations in regional myocardial distribution and arrhythmogenic effects of aprindine produced by coronary artery occlusion in the dog. Cardiovasc Res, 1981. **15**(2): pp. 80–5.

[90] Greenberg, H.M., et al., Interaction of ischaemia and encainide/flecainide treatment: a proposed mechanism for the increased mortality in CAST I. Br Heart J, 1995. **74**(6): pp. 631–5.

[91] Gottlieb, S.S. and M. Packer, Deleterious hemodynamic effects of lidocaine in severe congestive heart failure. Am Heart J, 1989. **118**(3): pp. 611–2.

[92] Gottlieb, S.S., et al., Comparative hemodynamic effects of procainamide, tocainide, and encainide in severe chronic heart failure. Circulation, 1990. **81**(3): pp. 860–4.

[93] Smith, D.I., et al., Trial ultrasound-guided continuous left stellate ganglion blockade before surgical gangliolysis in a patient with a left ventricular assist device and intractable ventricular tachycardia: a pain control application to a complex hemodynamic condition. ASAIO J, 2015. **61**(1): pp. 104–6.

[94] Collura, C.A., et al., Left cardiac sympathetic denervation for the treatment of long QT syndrome and catecholaminergic polymorphic ventricular tachycardia using video-assisted thoracic surgery. Heart Rhythm, 2009. **6**(6): pp. 752–9.

[95] Mahajan, A., et al., Use of thoracic epidural anesthesia for management of electrical storm: a case report. Heart Rhythm, 2005. **2**(12): pp. 1359–62.

[96] Blomberg, S., et al., Thoracic epidural anaesthesia in patients with unstable angina pectoris. Eur Heart J, 1989. **10**(5): pp. 437–44.

[97] Staats, P.S. and S.J. Panchal, Pro: the anesthesiologist should provide epidural anesthesia in the coronary care unit for patients with severe angina. J Cardiothorac Vasc Anesth, 1997. **11**(1): pp. 105–8.

[98] Loyalka, P., et al., Left stellate ganglion block for continuous ventricular arrhythmias during percutaneous left ventricular assist device support. Tex Heart Inst J, 2011. **38**(4): pp. 409–11.

[99] Malik, A.A., et al., Percutaneous inferior cervical sympathetic ganglion blockade for the treatment of ventricular tachycardia storm: case report and review of the literature. J Vasc Interv Neurol, 2014. **7**(5): pp. 48–51.

[100] Dowling, N.F., et al., The U.S. Thrombosis and Hemostasis Centers pilot sites program. J Thromb Thrombolysis, 2007. **23**(1): pp. 1–7.

[101] Schulman, S., et al., Hemorrhagic complications of anticoagulant and thrombolytic treatment: American College of Chest Physicians Evidence-Based Clinical Practice Guidelines (8th Edition). Chest, 2008. **133**(6 Suppl): pp. 257S–298.

[102] Li, J. and T. Halaszynski, Neuraxial and peripheral nerve blocks in patients taking anticoagulant or thromboprophylactic drugs: challenges and solutions. Local Reg Anesth, 2015. **8**: pp. 21–32.

[103] Gomez-Outes, A., et al., Pharmacoeconomic evaluation of dabigatran, rivaroxaban and apixaban versus enoxaparin for the prevention of venous thromboembolism after total hip or knee replacement in Spain. Pharmacoeconomics, 2014. **32**(9): pp. 919–36.

[104] Ladwig, K.H., et al., Absence of an impact of emotional distress on the perception of intracardiac shock discharges. Int J Behav Med, 2003. **10**(1): pp. 56–65.

[105] Glikson, M. and P.A. Friedman, The implantable cardioverter defibrillator. Lancet, 2001. **357**(9262): pp. 1107–17.

[106] Hammill, S.C., et al., Termination and acceleration of ventricular tachycardia with autodecremental pacing, burst pacing, and cardioversion in patients with an implantable cardioverter defibrillator. Multicenter PCD Investigator Group. Pacing Clin Electrophysiol, 1995. **18**(1 Pt 1): pp. 3–10.

[107] Fricchione, G.L., L.C. Olson, and S.C. Vlay, Psychiatric syndromes in patients with the automatic internal cardioverter defibrillator: anxiety, psychological dependence, abuse, and withdrawal. Am Heart J, 1989. **117**(6): pp. 1411–4.

[108] Hamner, M., et al., PTSD and automatic implantable cardioverter defibrillators. Psychosomatics, 1999. **40**(1): pp. 82–5.

[109] Sears, S.F., Jr., et al., Examining the psychosocial impact of implantable cardioverter defibrillators: a literature review. Clin Cardiol, 1999. **22**(7): pp. 481–9.

[110] Sears, S.F., Jr. and J.B. Conti, Quality of life and psychological functioning of icd patients. Heart, 2002. **87**(5): pp. 488–93.

[111] Schron, E.B., et al., Quality of life in the antiarrhythmics versus implantable defibrillators trial: impact of therapy and influence of adverse symptoms and defibrillator shocks. Circulation, 2002. **105**(5): pp. 589–94.

[112] Sowell, L.V., et al., Anxiety and marital adjustment in patients with implantable cardioverter defibrillator and their spouses. J Cardiopulm Rehabil Prev, 2007. **27**(1): pp. 46–9.

[113] Mark, D.B., et al., Quality of life with defibrillator therapy or amiodarone in heart failure. N Engl J Med, 2008. **359**(10): pp. 999–1008.

Section 2

Role of Implantable Devices in the Management of Systolic Heart Failure

Chapter 3

The Impact of Cardiac Resynchronization Therapy in the Treatment of Heart Failure

Takashi Murashita

Additional information is available at the end of the chapter

http://dx.doi.org/10.5772/66947

Abstract

The number of patients who suffer from heart failure is rapidly increasing. In about one-third of heart failure patients, conduction delays cause dyssynchronous left ventricular contractions, which leads to reduction in left ventricular function, adverse cardiac remodelling and finally increased mortality. Cardiac resynchronization involves simultaneous pacing of both ventricles, and improves left ventricular contractile function. Although resynchronization does not restore myocardial function, multiple studies have shown that cardiac resynchronization therapy improves quality of life, exercise capacity, symptoms of heart failure, left ventricular ejection fraction, morbidity and mortality. The use of cardiac resynchronization therapy has increased significantly, since its initial approval in 2001, in patients with advanced heart failure.

Keywords: heart failure, cardiac resynchronization therapy, electrophysiologist, left bundle branch block, left ventricular function

1. Introduction

The number of patients who suffer from chronic heart failure is rapidly growing. According to the 2016 update on heart disease and stroke statistics reported by the American Heart Association, an estimated 5.7 million Americans ≥20 years of age have a diagnosis of heart failure and projections show that the prevalence of heart failure will increase 46% from 2012 to 2030, resulting in >8 million people ≥18 years of age with heart failure [1]. In the year of 2013, heart failure was the underlying cause in >65,000 deaths and contributed to the death of >300,000 people [1]. In the same report, there is an estimate that a total cost of over $30 billion was used for the treatment of heart failure in 2012 [1]. Direct medical costs attributed to 68% of this total amount. The lifetime risk of developing heart failure is 20% for adults at the age of 40 years and goes up with age. Acute heart failure consists of one of the most common reasons for hospitalization, attributing to over 1 million discharges annually and high 30-day readmission rates (up to 25%) and 1 year (up to 60%) [1]. The prognosis for heart failure is poor, with an estimated mortality rate of 50% within 5 years of diagnosis.

2. Cardiac resynchronization therapy (CRT)

2.1. Advent of CRT

An intraventricular conduction delay is found in approximately 20–30% of patients with symptomatic heart failure. Conduction delay causes dyssynchronous left ventricular contractions, which lead to left ventricular dysfunction, adverse cardiac remodelling and eventually high mortality [2–4]. Conduction delay may also lead to mitral valve regurgitation, thus increasing symptoms of heart failure. The prevalence of left ventricular dyssynchrony in heart failure has been shown to increase with reduced left ventricular ejection fraction and with increased QRS width [5–7].

Cardiac resynchronization therapy (CRT), which was first introduced for clinical use in 1996, attempts to restore ventricular synchrony in patients who suffer from dilated cardiomyopathy with a widened QRS complex to improve the mechanical efficiency of left ventricular contraction. Since U.S. Food and Drug Administration (FDA) approval, the use of CRT has steadily increased [8]. Sridhar and colleagues showed a trend in CRT device implantation in the United States [9] (**Figure 1**).

2.2. Mechanism of CRT

Janaswamy et al. listed the studies which demonstrated that the presence of a bundle branch block or other intraventricular conduction delay can worsen heart failure due to systolic dysfunction by causing ventricular dyssynchrony [10] (**Table 1**). The rationale for CRT is based upon these findings. These acute mechanical benefits of CRT can be accompanied with more chronic adaptations that lead to long-term benefit in the patient who suffers from heart failure [11].

Nowadays, it has been reported that CRT improves quality of life, exercise capacity, symptoms of heart failure by [12–16] left ventricular ejection fraction [17, 18], morbidity and mortality [18] in patients with moderate to severe left ventricular dysfunction with a wide QRS complex. The benefit of CRT in mild to moderate heart failure has also been demonstrated by several studies [19–23]. Long-term beneficial effects on left ventricular function were shown by positron emission tomography evaluations, and CRT enhances myocardial forward work efficiency at rest in patients with dilated cardiomyopathy and heart failure [24, 25].

CRT improves left ventricular contractile function in patients with heart failure associated with left bundle branch block. Improved efficiency from resynchronization pacing is unlikely due to the alterations in intrinsic myocyte function. The improvement of ventricular function is the result of improved efficiency of the work performed by different regions of the wall. Nelson et al. demonstrated that pressure-volume loops display an increase in loop area and width (stroke work and volume, respectively) and a decline in end systolic volume with

http://dx.doi.org/10.5772/66947

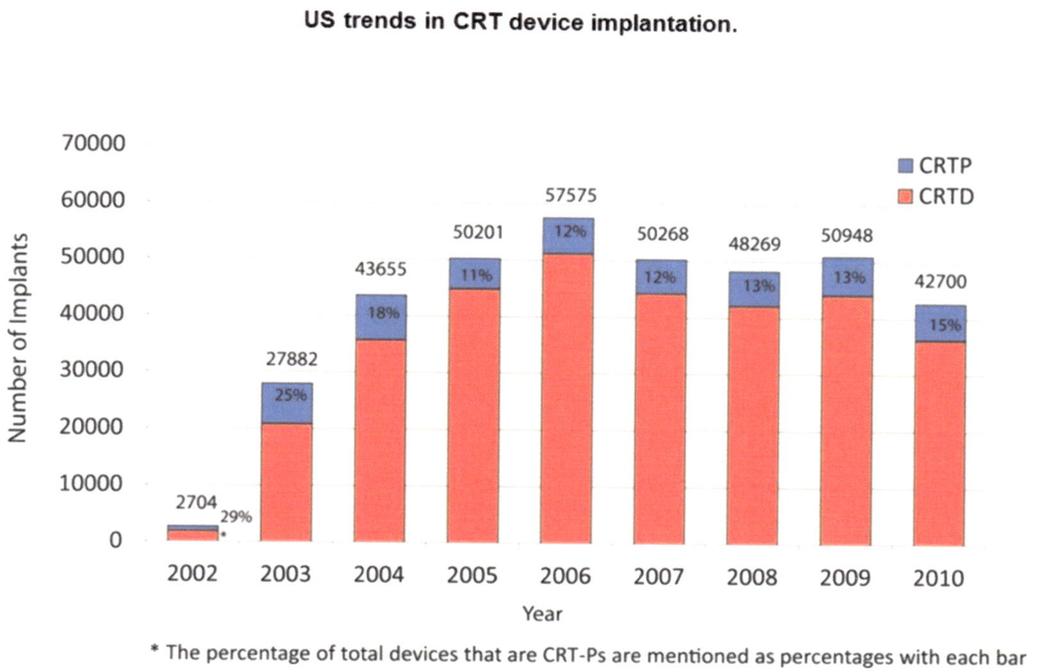

Figure 1. The number of CRT device implantation in the United States.

pacing [25]. In spite of improvements in systolic function, myocardial oxygen consumption decreases due to a slight fall in coronary flow as well as transcardiac oxygen gradient.

2.3. U.S. trends in CRT

CRT is now recommended for patients with heart failure due to systolic dysfunction combined with intraventricular delay. CRT is also recommended in addition to guideline-directed medical therapy, such as angiotensin-converting enzyme inhibitors, beta blockers, aldosterone antagonist therapy and implantable cardioverter defibrillators (ICDs) when indicated for primary or secondary prevention of sudden cardiac death.

Sridhar et al. used the Nationwide Inpatient Sample database to identify all patients who underwent CRT implantation during 2002–2010 [9]. The overall trends in CRT device implantation, patient characteristics and outcomes were studied in detail and comparisons among demographic subgroups were performed. They found that an average of 41,578 CRT device implantations was performed per year. There has been a significant increase in the percentage of CRTs implanted in patients with advanced age (≥85 years). There were significant differences in CRT utilization favouring male and whites compared with female and black patients, respectively, in spite of adjustments for rates of heart failure. The highest numbers of implants were found in the patient group with moderate comorbidity (48%), followed by mild comorbidity group (39/7%). The overall number of CRT implantations in the severe comorbidity group was the lowest (12.3%). However, in the recent years, there has been a significant increase in the number of CRT implantation in this category (**Figure 2**).

Trial	Inclusion criteria	Primary end point	Follow-up	Results/conclusion
MIRACLE [12]	QRS duration ≥130 ms, an LV end diastolic diameter ≥55 mm by echocardiography and ejection fraction (EF) ≤0.35	NYHA symptom class, quality of life (Minnesota Living with heart failure questionnaire) and exercise capacity	6 months	Significant reductions in LVEDV ($P < 0.001$) and LVESV ($P < 0.001$) at 3 months, and continued to 6 months, in the CRT group compared with the control group. Significant improvement in EF compared with the control group at 3 months (2.3 vs. 0.6%; $P < 0.01$) and 6 months (3.6 vs. 0.4%; $P < 0.001$). Significant decrease in severity of MR at 3 months (-2.1 vs. 0.1 cm^2 jet area; $P < 0.01$) and at 6 months (-2.5 vs. 0.5 cm^2 jet area; $P < 0.001$). Increase in cardiac index from baseline to 6 months (0.11 L · min-1 · m-2; $P < 0.05$).
PATH-CHF [13]	NYHA functional class III or IV, dilated cardiomyopathy of any etiology, sinus rhythm ≥55 beats/min, a QRS complex duration ≥120 ms in at least two surface electrocardiographic (ECG) leads and a PR interval ≥150 ms	Primary end points: oxygen uptake at peak exercise, oxygen uptake at the anaerobic threshold and the 6-min walking distance. The secondary end points were changes in NYHA functional class and quality of life.	12 months	Oxygen uptake during bicycle exercise increased from 9.48 to 10.4 ml/kg/min at the anaerobic threshold ($P = 0.03$) and from 12.5 to 14.3 ml/kg/min at peak exercise ($P < 0.001$) with the first treatment. From 10.0 to 10.7 ml/kg/min at the anaerobic threshold ($P = 0.2$) and from 13.4 to 15.2 ml/kg/min at peak exercise ($P = 0.002$) with the second treatment. Increase in maximal exercise capacity from 12.6 to 15.6 ml/kg/min. Increase in 6-min walk performance from 357 to 466 m. 2/3 of patients improved to NYHA functional class I or II.
MUSTIC [14]	Severe HF with EF < 0.35 as measured by radionuclides and an LV end diastolic diameter >60 mm NYHA functional class III. The 6-min walking distance <450 m. QRS duration >150 ms. AF > 3 months. QRS duration >200 ms	6-min walking distance, the peak VO2 by cardiopulmonary exercise test, quality of life, NYHA class, systolic and diastolic blood pressure (BP), body weight, 12-lead surface electrocardiogram (ECG), 24-h Holter monitoring and Doppler echocardiography	1 year	Significant improvement in 6-min walk distance of 20% compared with baseline at 6, 9 and 12 months. Peak VO2 at 12 months had increased by 1.7 ml/min/kg or 11% in the SR group and 1.1 ml/kg/min or 9% in the AF group compared with baseline. Reduction in the Minnesota score of 17 points or 36% in the SR group and of 14 points or 32% in the AF group. The NYHA class improved by 0.7 in the SR group and 0.8 in the AF group.

Trial	Inclusion criteria	Primary end point	Follow-up	Results/conclusion
MIRACLE ICD [16] Combination with ICD	Cardiac arrest due to VF or VT, or spontaneously sustained ventricular tachyarrhythmia, or inducible ventricular fibrillation or sustained ventricular tachyarrhythmia, NYHA III or IV LVEF ≤ 0.35 QRS duration ≥130 ms LVEDD ≥55 mm	Primary end points: NYHA functional class, quality-of-life score and distance covered during the 6-min walking test.	1, 3 and 6 months.	Significantly higher median improvement in quality of life, NYHA functional class and distance during 6-min walk in the CRT group compared with the control group.
RAFT [19] ICD + CRT	NHYA class II or III, EF <0.30, an intrinsic QRS duration of 120 ms or more or a paced QRS duration of 200 ms or more, sinus rhythm or permanent AF or flutter with a controlled ventricular rate (≤60 beats per minute at rest and ≤90 beats per minute during a 6-min walk test) or planned atrioventricular-junction ablation after device implantation), and planned ICD implantation for indicated primary or secondary prevention of sudden cardiac death	Primary outcome: death from any cause or heart failure leading to hospitalization	The mean (±SD) follow-up period was 40 ± 20 months for all patients and 44 ± 18 months for surviving patients	Prolonged time to the occurrence of the primary outcome in the ICD–CRT group (hazard ratio, 0.75; 95% confidence interval [CI], 0.64–0.87; $P < 0.001$). The time until death was significantly prolonged (relative risk reduction, 25%) in the ICD–CRT group (hazard ratio, 0.75; 95% CI, 0.62–0.91; $P = 0.003$).
COMPANION [29] Pharmacologic therapy alone, pharmacologic + CRV with pacemaker, pharmacologic + CRT+ pacemaker defibrillator	NYHA class III or IV HF, LVEF of 0.35 or less, QRS interval of at least 120 ms and a PR interval of more than 150 ms, sinus rhythm, no clinical indication for a pacemaker or ICD, and a hospitalization for the treatment of heart failure or the equivalent in the preceding 12 months.	primary end point: composite of death from any cause or hospitalization for any cause	Median duration of follow-up for the primary end point: 11.9 months in the pharmacologic therapy group, 16.2 months in the pacemaker group and 15.7 months in the pacemaker defibrillator group	12-month rate of death from any cause or hospitalization for any cause was 68% in the pharmacologic therapy group as compared with 56% in the pacemaker group (hazard ratio for the primary end point: 0.81) and 56% in the pacemaker defibrillator group (hazard ratio, 0.80)

Trial	Inclusion criteria	Primary end point	Follow-up	Results/conclusion
MADIT-CRT [30] ICD and CRT	Ejection fraction of 30% or less, a QRS duration of 130 ms or more, and NYHA class I or II symptoms	Death from any cause or nonfatal heart failure events, whichever came first	Follow-up of patients in the trial averaged 2.4 years	34% reduction in the risk of death or nonfatal heart failure (whichever came first) among patients in the CRT–ICD group, as compared with those in the ICD-only group. CRT–ICD therapy was associated with a greater benefit in women (hazard ratio, 0.37; 95% confidence interval [CI], 0.22–0.61) than in men (hazard ratio, 0.76; 95% CI, 0.59–0.97; $P = 0.01$ for interaction) and in patients with a QRS duration of 150 ms or more (hazard ratio, 0.48; 95% CI, 0.37–0.64) than in those with a QRS duration of less than 150 ms (hazard ratio, 1.06; 95% CI, 0.74–1.52; $P = 0.001$ for interaction).
REVERSE [31]	QRS ≥120 ms and LV ejection fraction ≤0.40, active 55-mm or wider LV end diastolic diameter, measured by echocardiography	Primary end point: HF clinical composite response	Patients were followed at 1, 3, 6, 12, 18 and 24 months	Worsening of the HF clinical composite response in 34 of the 180 patients (19%) assigned to CRT ON compared with 28 of the 82 patients (34%) assigned to CRT OFF ($p = 0.01$). LVESVi decreased by a mean of 27.5 ± 31.8 ml/m2 in the CRT ON compared with 2.7 ± 25.8 ml/m2 in the CRT OFF group ($P < 0.0001$). Rates of HF hospital stay was 14 of 82 (17.1%) in CRT OFF patients and 13 of 180 (7.2%) CRT ON patients

Table 1. Summary of studies of CRT.

2.4. Outcomes of CRT implantation

The in-hospital mortality rates associated with CRT implantation is shown in **Figure 3**.

For an elective CRT procedure, the mean length of stay was 2.81 days and the median was 1.00 day. The overall in-hospital mortality following CRT implantation was 0.87%, which has decreased significantly from 2003 to 2010 (1.08 in 2003 to 0.70% in 2010; $P = 0.03$). Mortality following elective CRT implantation was 0.4% compared with 1.0% with non-elective CRT implantations. The mortality was higher in male (0.93%) compared with female (0.71%), and decrease in mortality was observed in both male and female. The mortality rate in advanced age group (≥85 years) was significantly higher compared with younger population (<85 years). However, the mortality rate in the ≥85-year group has significantly decreased in recent years. Patients with

http://dx.doi.org/10.5772/66947

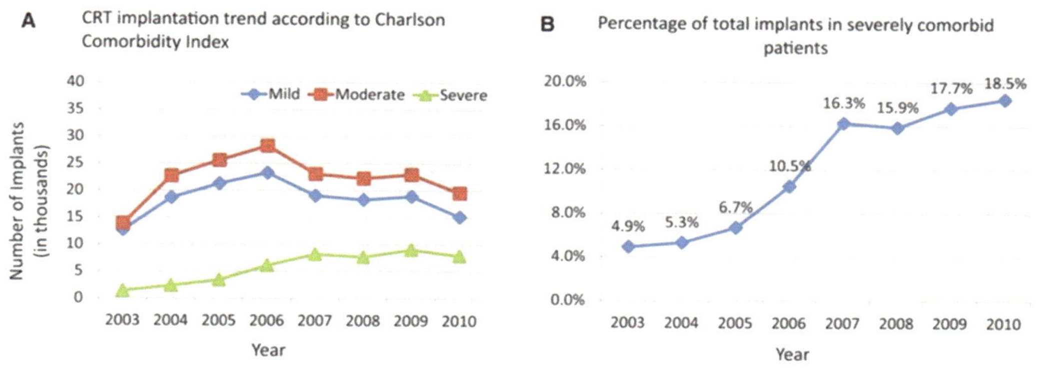

Figure 2. Patient comorbidities and CRT implantation. (A) CRT implantation trends stratified according to comorbidity categories. (B) CRT devices implanted in patients with severe comorbidities, expressed as a percentage of total CRT implants in the United States in each year.

severe comorbidities had significantly higher overall mortality (1.5%) compared with those with moderate (0.8%) or mild (0.7%) comorbidities ($P < 0.001$). However, mortality in all three comorbidity groups has decreased in recent years, most notably in the severe comorbidity group.

In terms of complications associated with CRT implantation, pericardial effusion was found in 0.2%, pneumothorax was found in 1.4% and hematoma was found in 3.0% of all CRT implantation procedures.

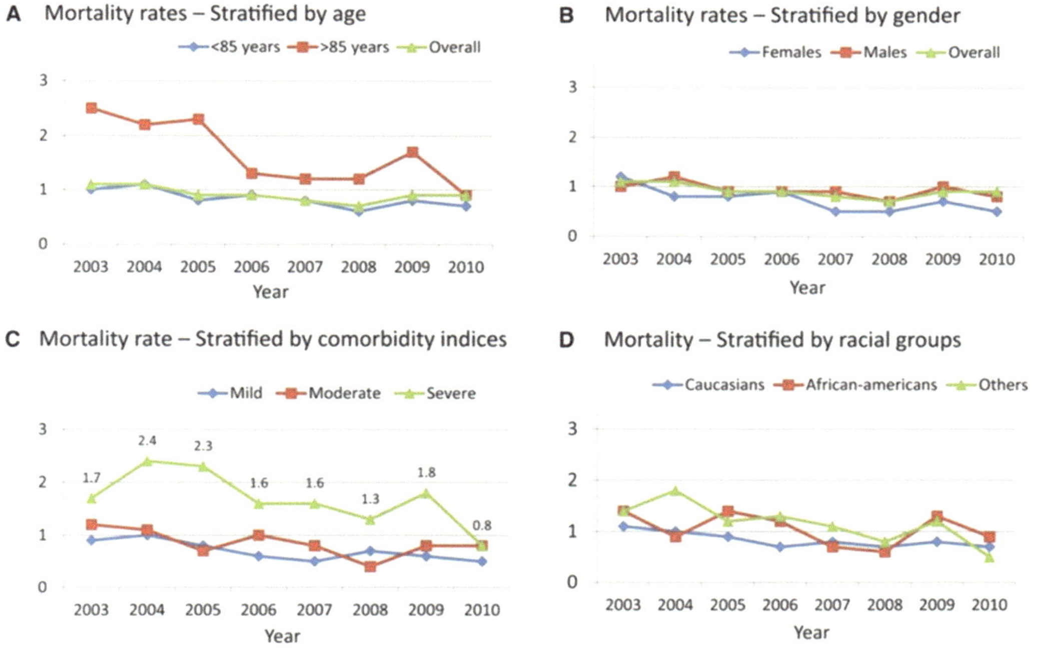

Figure 3. In-hospital mortality rates associated with CRT implantation stratified by patient characteristics.

The overall mean hospital charges accompanied with CRT implantation were reported to be $129,098 per implant. Of note, hospital charges for CRT implantation have dramatically increased from $111,197 in 2003 to $154,297 in 2010 ($P < 0.001$). Charges accompanied with CRT implantation were higher in male sex, ≥85-year group, and higher comorbidities compared with female sex, <85-year group, and lower comorbidities, respectively.

2.5. Implantation technique of CRT

Electrophysiologists are the main players for the CRT implantation. The CRT implantation requires the placement of a left ventricular pacing lead, which is fed onto the epicardial surface through a venous branch of the coronary sinus (**Figure 4**). Difficulty with coronary sinus cannulation, challenging anatomy of coronary sinus venous tributaries, unacceptable pacing and sensing thresholds, unavoidable phrenic nerve pacing and lead dislodgement have resulted in a 10–20% failure rate associated with left ventricular lead placement [16, 26]. When a transvenous lead implantation at desired sites is not achievable, epicardial left ventricular leads can easily be placed surgically directly on the lateral or posterolateral wall. Garikipati et al. performed a randomized study and reported no difference in the echocardiographic and clinical outcomes comparing a conventional transvenous approach versus surgical epicardial left ventricular lead placement for CRT [27]. Therefore, surgical approaches are a viable alternative when a transvenous procedure has failed or is not feasible.

Zhang et al. reported that advanced age, male sex, ischemic cause, end-stage heart failure, inadequate electrical delay and absence of mechanical dyssynchrony are regarded as non-modifiable risk factors for CRT non-responders [28]. However, efforts should be made to correct modifiable factors, such as suboptimal medical therapy, uncontrolled atrial fibrillation, left ventricular lead dislodgement or inappropriate location, loss of biventricular capture and lack of device optimization.

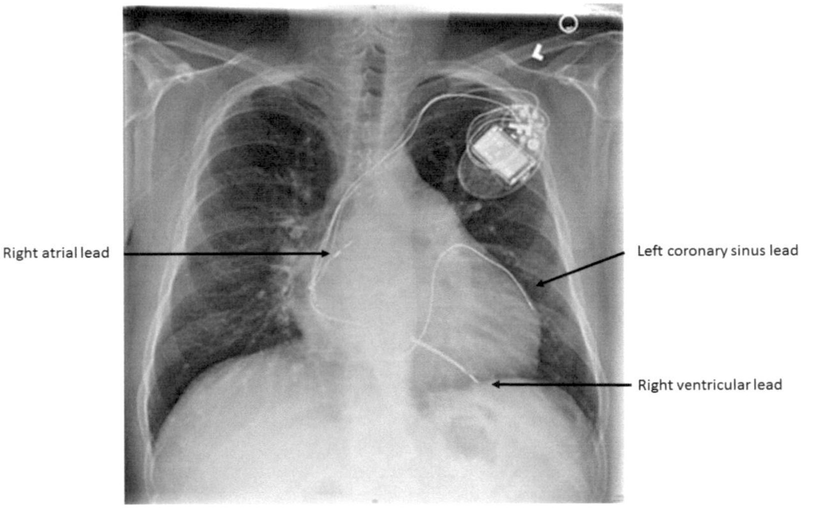

Figure 4. A chest X-ray after a successful CRT implantation.

3. Conclusions

CRT implantation is a safe procedure that has become safer in higher risk patients. With the increase of heart failure patients, CRT plays more and more role in the treatment of heart failure. Electrophysiologists should understand the indication, outcomes and procedure technique of CRT implantation.

Author details

Takashi Murashita

Address all correspondence to: tmurashita@gmail.com

Heart and Vascular Institute, West Virginia University, Morgantown, WV, USA

References

[1] Writing Group Members, Mozaffarian D, Benjamin EJ, Go AS, Arnett DK, Blaha MJ, Cushman M, Das SR, de Ferranti S, Després JP, Fullerton HJ, Howard VJ, Huffman MD, Isasi CR, Jiménez MC, Judd SE, Kissela BM, Lichtman JH, Lisabeth LD, Liu S, Mackey RH, Magid DJ, McGuire DK, Mohler ER 3rd, Moy CS, Muntner P, Mussolino ME, Nasir K, Neumar RW, Nichol G, Palaniappan L, Pandey DK, Reeves MJ, Rodriguez CJ, Rosamond W, Sorlie PD, Stein J, Towfighi A, Turan TN, Virani SS, Woo D, Yeh RW, Turner MB; American Heart Association Statistics Committee; Stroke Statistics Subcommittee. Heart disease and stroke statistics-2016 update: a report from the American heart association. Circulation. 2016;**133**(4):38–360. DOI: 10.1161/CIR.0000000000000350

[2] Baldasseroni S, Opasich C, Gorini M, Lucci D, Marchionni N, Marini M, Campana C, Perini G, Deorsola A, Masotti G, Tavazzi L, Maggioni AP; Italian Network on Congestive Heart Failure Investigators. Left bundle-branch block is associated with increased 1-year sudden and total mortality rate in 5517 outpatients with congestive heart failure: a report from the Italian network on congestive heart failure. Am Heart J. 2002;**143**(3):398–405.

[3] Kawaguchi M, Murabayashi T, Fetics BJ, Nelson GS, Samejima H, Nevo E, Kass DA. Quantitation of basal dyssynchrony and acute resynchronization from left or biventricular pacing by novel echo-contrast variability imaging. J Am Coll Cardiol. 2002;**39**(12):2052–8.

[4] Shamim W, Francis DP, Yousufuddin M, Varney S, Pieopli MF, Anker SD, Coats AJ. Intraventricular conduction delay: a prognostic marker in chronic heart failure. Int J Cardiol. 1999;**70**(2):171–8.

[5] De Sutter J, Van de Veire NR, Muyldermans L, De Backer T, Hoffer E, Vaerenberg M, Paelinck B, Decoodt P, Gabriel L, Gillebert TC, Van Camp G; Working Group of

Echocardiography and Cardiac Doppler of the Belgian Society of Cardiology. Prevalence of mechanical dyssynchrony in patients with heart failure and preserved left ventricular function (a report from the Belgian multicenter registry on dyssynchrony). Am J Cardiol. 2005;**96**(11):1543–8.

[6] Ghio S, Constantin C, Klersy C, Serio A, Fontana A, Campana C, Tavazzi L. Interventricular and intraventricular dyssynchrony are common in heart failure patients, regardless of QRS duration. Eur Heart J. 2004;**25**(7):571–8.

[7] Haghjoo M, Bagherzadeh A, Fazelifar AF, Haghighi ZO, Esmaielzadeh M, Alizadeh A, Emkanjoo Z, Sadeghpour A, Samiei N, Farahani MM, Sadr-Ameli MA, Maleki M, Noohi F. Prevalence of mechanical dyssynchrony in heart failure patients with different QRS durations. Pacing Clin Electrophysiol. 2007;**30**(5):616–22.

[8] Moynahan M, Faris OP, Lewis BM. Cardiac resynchronization devices: the Food and Drug Administration's regulatory considerations. J Am Coll Cardiol. 2005;**46**(12):2325–8.

[9] Sridhar AR, Yarlagadda V, Parasa S, Reddy YM, Patel D, Lakkireddy D, Wilkoff BL, Dawn B. Cardiac resynchronization therapy: US trends and disparities in utilization and outcomes. Circ Arrhythm Electrophysiol. 2016;**9**(e003108):26921376. DOI: 10.1161/CIRCEP.115.003108

[10] Janaswamy P, Walters TE, Nazer B, Lee RJ. Current treatment strategies for heart failure: role of device therapy and lv reconstruction. Curr Treat Options Cardiovasc Med. 2016;**18**(9):57. DOI: 10.1007/s11936-016-0479-1

[11] Abraham WT, Hayes DL. Cardiac resynchronization therapy for heart failure. Circulation. 2003;**108**(21):2596–603.

[12] Abraham WT, Fisher WG, Smith AL, Delurgio DB, Leon AR, Loh E, Kocovic DZ, Packer M, Clavell AL, Hayes DL, Ellestad M, Trupp RJ, Underwood J, Pickering F, Truex C, McAtee P, Messenger J; MIRACLE Study Group. Multicenter InSync randomized clinical evaluation. Cardiac resynchronization in chronic heart failure. N Engl J Med. 2002;**346**(24):1845–53.

[13] Auricchio A, Stellbrink C, Sack S, Block M, Vogt J, Bakker P, Huth C, Schöndube F, Wolfhard U, Böcker D, Krahnefeld O, Kirkels H; Pacing Therapies in Congestive Heart Failure (PATH-CHF) Study Group. Long-term clinical effect of hemodynamically optimized cardiac resynchronization therapy in patients with heart failure and ventricular conduction delay. J Am Coll Cardiol. 2002;**39**(12):2026–33.

[14] Cazeau S, Leclercq C, Lavergne T, Walker S, Varma C, Linde C, Garrigue S, Kappenberger L, Haywood GA, Santini M, Bailleul C, Daubert JC; Multisite Stimulation in Cardiomyopathies (MUSTIC) Study Investigators. Effects of multisite biventricular pacing in patients with heart failure and intraventricular conduction delay. N Engl J Med. 2001;**344**(12):873–80.

[15] Higgins SL, Hummel JD, Niazi IK, Giudici MC, Worley SJ, Saxon LA, Boehmer JP, Higginbotham MB, De Marco T, Foster E, Yong PG. Cardiac resynchronization therapy

http://dx.doi.org/10.5772/66947

for the treatment of heart failure in patients with intraventricular conduction delay and malignant ventricular tachyarrhythmias. J Am Coll Cardiol. 2003;**42**(8):1454–9.

[16] Young JB, Abraham WT, Smith AL, Leon AR, Lieberman R, Wilkoff B, Canby RC, Schroeder JS, Liem LB, Hall S, Wheelan K; Multicenter InSync ICD Randomized Clinical Evaluation (MIRACLE ICD) Trial Investigators. Combined cardiac resynchronization and implantable cardioversion defibrillation in advanced chronic heart failure: the MIRACLE ICD Trial. JAMA. 2003;**289**(20):2685–94.

[17] Sutton MG, Plappert T, Hilpisch KE, Abraham WT, Hayes DL, Chinchoy E. Sustained reverse left ventricular structural remodeling with cardiac resynchronization at one year is a function of etiology: quantitative Doppler echocardiographic evidence from the Multicenter InSync randomized clinical evaluation (MIRACLE). Circulation. 2006;**113**(2):266–72.

[18] Cleland JG, Daubert JC, Erdmann E, Freemantle N, Gras D, Kappenberger L, Tavazzi L; Cardiac Resynchronization-Heart Failure (CARE-HF) Study Investigators. The effect of cardiac resynchronization on morbidity and mortality in heart failure. N Engl J Med. 2005;**352**(15):1539–49.

[19] Tang AS, Wells GA, Talajic M, Arnold MO, Sheldon R, Connolly S, Hohnloser SH, Nichol G, Birnie DH, Sapp JL, Yee R, Healey JS, Rouleau JL; Resynchronization-Defibrillation for Ambulatory Heart Failure Trial Investigators. Cardiac-resynchronization therapy for mild-to-moderate heart failure. N Engl J Med. 2010;**363**(25):2385–95.

[20] Moss AJ, Hall WJ, Cannom DS, Klein H, Brown MW, Daubert JP, Estes NA 3rd, Foster E, Greenberg H, Higgins SL, Pfeffer MA, Solomon SD, Wilber D, Zareba W; MADIT-CRT Trial Investigators. Cardiac-resynchronization therapy for the prevention of heart-failure events. N Engl J Med. 2009;**361**(14):1329–38.

[21] Linde C, Abraham WT, Gold MR, St John Sutton M, Ghio S, Daubert C; REVERSE (REsynchronization reVErses Remodeling in Systolic left vEntricular dysfunction) Study Group. Randomized trial of cardiac resynchronization in mildly symptomatic heart failure patients and in asymptomatic patients with left ventricular dysfunction and previous heart failure symptoms. J Am Coll Cardiol. 2008;**52**(23):1834–43.

[22] Abraham WT, Young JB, León AR, Adler S, Bank AJ, Hall SA, Lieberman R, Liem LB, O'Connell JB, Schroeder JS, Wheelan KR; Multicenter InSync ICD II Study Group. Effects of cardiac resynchronization on disease progression in patients with left ventricular systolic dysfunction, an indication for an implantable cardioverter-defibrillator, and mildly symptomatic chronic heart failure. Circulation. 2004;**110**(18):2864–8.

[23] Veazie PJ, Noyes K, Li Q, Hall WJ, Buttaccio A, Thevenet-Morrison K, Moss AJ. Cardiac resynchronization and quality of life in patients with minimally symptomatic heart failure. J Am Coll Cardiol. 2012;**60**(19):1940–4.

[24] Ukkonen H, Beanlands RS, Burwash IG, de Kemp RA, Nahmias C, Fallen E, Hill MR, Tang AS. Effect of cardiac resynchronization on myocardial efficiency and regional oxidative metabolism. Circulation. 2003;**107**(1):28–31.

[25] Nelson GS, Berger RD, Fetics BJ, Talbot M, Spinelli JC, Hare JM, Kass DA. Left ventricular or biventricular pacing improves cardiac function at diminished energy cost in patients with dilated cardiomyopathy and left bundle-branch block. Circulation. 2000;**102**(25):3053–9.

[26] Mullens W, Grimm RA, Verga T, Dresing T, Starling RC, Wilkoff BL, Tang WH. Insights from a cardiac resynchronization optimization clinic as part of a heart failure disease management program. J Am Coll Cardiol. 2009;**53**(9):765–73. DOI: 10.1016/j.jacc.2008.11.024

[27] Garikipati NV, Mittal S, Chaudhry F, Musat DL, Sichrovsky T, Preminger M, Arshad A, Steinberg JS. Comparison of endovascular versus epicardial lead placement for resynchronization therapy. Am J Cardiol. 2014;**113**(5):840–4. DOI: 10.1016/j.amjcard.2013.11.040

[28] Zhang Q, Zhou Y, Yu CM. Incidence, definition, diagnosis, and management of the cardiac resynchronization therapy nonresponder. Curr Opin Cardiol. 2015;**30**(1):40–9. DOI: 10.1097/HCO.0000000000000140

[29] Bristow MR, Saxon LA, Boehmer J, Krueger S, Kass DA, De Marco T, Carson P, DiCarlo L, DeMets D, White BG, DeVries DW, Feldman AM; Comparison of Medical Therapy, Pacing, and Defibrillation in Heart Failure (COMPANION) Investigators. Cardiac-resynchronization therapy with or without an implantable defibrillator in advanced chronic heart failure. N Engl J Med. 2004;**350**(21):2140–50.

[30] Zareba W, Klein H, Cygankiewicz I, Hall WJ, McNitt S, Brown M, Cannom D, Daubert JP, Eldar M, Gold MR, Goldberger JJ, Goldenberg I, Lichstein E, Pitschner H, Rashtian M, Solomon S, Viskin S, Wang P, Moss AJ; MADIT-CRT Investigators. Effectiveness of cardiac resynchronization therapy by QRS morphology in the multicenter automatic defibrillator implantation trial-cardiac resynchronization therapy (MADIT-CRT). Circulation. 2011;**123**(10):1061–72. DOI: 10.1161/CIRCULATIONAHA.110.960898

[31] Daubert C, Gold MR, Abraham WT, Ghio S, Hassager C, Goode G, Szili-Török T, Linde C; REVERSE Study Group. Prevention of disease progression by cardiac resynchronization therapy in patients with asymptomatic or mildly symptomatic left ventricular dysfunction: insights from the European cohort of the REVERSE (Resynchronization reverses remodeling in systolic left ventricular dysfunction) trial. J Am Coll Cardiol. 2009;**54**(20):1837–46. DOI: 10.1016/j.jacc.2009.08.011

Chapter 4

Cardiac Resynchronization Therapy in Advanced Heart Failure: Predictors of Response and Optimization of Therapy

García García Miguel Ángel,
Martínez Cornejo Alfonso and
Rosero Arenas María de los Ángeles

Additional information is available at the end of the chapter

http://dx.doi.org/10.5772/64611

Abstract

Heart failure affects a high percentage of the population, especially older patients. Cardiac resynchronization therapy is indicated in some patients with advanced heart failure. However, 20–40% of patients with implanted resynchronization device have no clinical response. In this chapter, we review factors related with the absence of a clinical response, recent technological advances that can reduce the failure rate, and an algorithm for management of patients without a clinical response.

Keywords: heart failure, cardiac resynchronization therapy, predictors of response to resynchronization, optimization of resynchronization, resynchronization-nonresponder-patients

1. Background

Heart failure affects more than 23 million people worldwide (2.4% of the adult population, with 11% that is older than 80 years) [1]. Its prevalence is increasing in recent years. It is a progressive disease, and its two leading causes of death are progressive heart failure and sudden death due to arrhythmia [2]. In an advanced stage of heart failure, patients have a limitation of their daily activity, frequent hospital admissions and medical treatment only slows the evolution of the disease. Cardiac resynchronization therapy (CRT) is indicated in some of these patients [3, 4].

2. Predictors of response to cardiac resynchronization therapy

Cardiac resynchronization is indicated in patients with heart failure, systolic dysfunction, and prolonged QRS interval since it could decrease mortality in this group of patients. Unfortunately, up to 40% do not experience clinical improvement to this therapy. **Table 1** shows the probable causes of this absence of response.

—	Presence of a large myocardial scar
—	Progressive heart failure
—	Noncompliance with pharmacological treatment
—	Not properly treated comorbidities (anemia, renal failure)
—	Suboptimal positioning of the electrodes
—	Suboptimal device programming
—	Absence of left ventricular dyssynchrony
—	Phrenic nerve stimulation

Table 1. Causes of the absence of response to cardiac resynchronization.

The prevalence of heart failure is higher in older patients. Many diseases show a lower response to treatment in older patients. Also, these older patients are usually excluded from clinical trials. The results of studies showing the effect of cardiac resynchronization therapy in elderly patients are contradictory. Some studies [5] do not show differences in mortality in older and younger patients. Other works [6] show that a greater age is a risk factor for higher mortality, together with other data (New York Heart Association functional class IV, impaired renal function, atrial fibrillation, and left ventricular ejection fraction <22%). With this doubt, the implantation of these devices could be considered in patients with advanced functional stages and older age.

Factors such as ischemic heart disease, monomorphic ventricular tachycardia, and the presence of moderate-to-severe mitral regurgitation have been associated with a decreased response to CRT [7].

The patients' baseline ECG, prior to implantation, also provides data that may help predict the response to resynchronization. The presence of a left bundle branch block (unlike right bundle branch block or other intraventricular conduction disorders) [8], atrial fibrillation, and a prolonged QRS interval is a factor related to a positive response to resynchronization treatment. The width of the QRS interval is another element to be evaluated. A QRS of 120–140 ms often occurs in left ventricular hypertrophy rather than in a true complete left bundle branch block; thus, the complete left bundle block is redefined as a QRS width >140 ms in men and >130 ms in women. A longer intraventricular conduction time is associated with a greater probability of echocardiographic inverse remodeling. An inverse relationship between QRS interval width and risk of death has been described [9]; in patients with QRS ≥145 ms, there is a benefit in survival, and there is no survival benefit in patients with ≤130 ms. Thus, according to the recent guidelines [3], cardiac resynchronization is not recommended in patients with narrow QRS.

The presence of atrial fibrillation or atrial conduction delay is associated with a lower response to resynchronization; this second problem could be corrected with electrical activation with an electrode at the interatrial septum [8].

A 12-lead ECG recorded following implantation of a CRT device may also predict one's response to resynchronization therapy. Optimal biventricular pacing, which coordinates the systolic activity of the interventricular septum and free walls of the left ventricle, may be realized as a tall R wave (>0.4 mm) in lead V1 with a predominantly negative deflection in I (RV1SI pattern) and is accompanied by improvement in heart failure and a lower mortality [10, 11]. An increase in the size of the R wave in V1 and the deviation of the QRS from the right to the left in relation to baseline ECG is associated with lower left ventricular systolic volumes. The decrease of the width of the non-paced QRS complex after initiation of resynchronization, or electrical remodeling, may also be associated with a lower risk of ventricular arrhythmias and lower mortality [12, 13]. Despite the above criteria, there is no clear relationship between mechanical and electrical remodeling.

Several case reports have exposed the detriment of selecting an inappropriate candidate for CRT device insertion. Investigators have described [14] the clinical course of a patient with a dilated cardiomyopathy, narrow QRS with anterosuperior hemiblock pattern, advanced heart failure, and absence of dyssynchrony. The implantation of a CRT device was followed by a widening of the QRS complex, since pacing of the right ventricle did not achieve adequate fusion with the ventricular complex itself and worsened heart failure. The patient's clinical status improved by optimizing the atrioventricular delay, resulting in a narrowing of the QRS complex. It is very difficult to select resynchronization candidates only by echocardiographic asynchrony or by wide QRS.

The interrogation of the device can provide several abnormal pacing data: defective implantation or failure of capture of the left ventricular electrode, delayed ventricular electrical conduction due to ventricular disease, or fusion beats between paced and spontaneous beats [10]. Electrophysiologists can correct some alterations, for example, by shortening atrioventricular delay or by varying the pacing interval between left and right ventricle. Pseudofusion, or ventricular pacing that start simultaneously with native complexes, and ineffective pacing, may be alleviated in part with medication that increases atrioventricular block or even with atrioventricular node ablation.

Heart failure is a progressive disease; however, stabilization of the clinic course may indicate a positive response to CRT. CRT nonresponders exhibit a progressive worsening of their heart failure (**Figure 1**), following device implantation. On the other end of the spectrum are the super-responders, who exhibit a significant improvement in the echocardiographic parameters of heart failure (100% increase of the left ventricular ejection fraction, or a final value of this parameter of at least 45%, 12 months after the implantation). The most frequently observed characteristics associated with the super-responders are extreme intraventricular conduction delays with QRS width ≥150 ms, typically with a complete left bundle branch block, female gender, non-ischemic cardiomyopathy, lower body mass index, and a smaller left atrial size [15, 16]. These data may help to screen patients who will reap the greatest benefit associated with resynchronization therapy, although the necessary optimization of the medical treatment of heart failure cannot be forgotten.

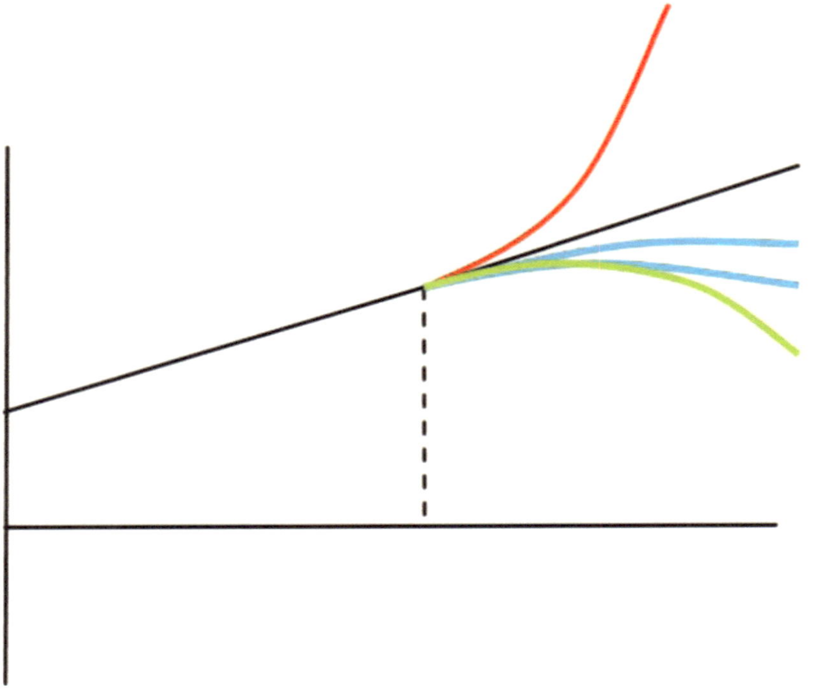

Figure 1. Graphical representation of the progression of heart failure (ordinates) as a function of time (abscissa). Dotted line, time of implantation of the resynchronization device; red line, negative responder; black line, nonresponder; blue lines, responders; green line, super-responder.

CRT devices may delay the need for a left ventricular assist device, in patients with advanced cardiac failure, who are hospitalized in need with inotropic support [17]. There may be up to 16% of response rate, especially in those patients with a complete left bundle branch block and a smaller left atrium.

3. Relationship between mechanical and electrical resynchronization

The concepts of mechanical and electrical remodeling refer to two distinct concepts: the first one is the mechanical improvement of the heart, and the second one is the electrical changes that tend to produce a less variegated electrical pattern.

This mechanical remodeling of the heart has already been observed previously in patients with optimal treatment for heart failure. Cardiac resynchronization produces a level of inverse

http://dx.doi.org/10.5772/64611

echocardiographic remodeling added to that achieved with appropriate pharmacologic therapy [18]. On an anatomopathologic level, there is a decrease in the degree of myocardial fibrosis [19].

Previous investigators have described how intraventricular conduction delay causes dyssynchronous cardiac contraction [18], with mechanical asynchrony (obtained by tissue Doppler) and delayed electrical activation of the left ventricular free wall. This has been observed in patients with a dilated cardiomyopathy, poor left ventricular function, and a complete left bundle branch block. However, many studies have shown a poor correlation between echocardiographic and electrographic data [20]. The PROSPECT study [21] showed that standard measures performed with conventional echocardiography do not distinguish between responders and nonresponders to CRT. Therefore, echocardiographic parameters were not useful in predicting clinical response. Studies using real-time three-dimensional echocardiography attempted to improve discrimination as compared to conventional 2D echocardiography, and found the systolic dysincrony index, a parameter that evaluates ventricular hemodynamics globally and may help predict changes in hemodynamics with a sensitivity greater than 80% [22].

Cardiac dyssynchrony has also been described in patients who have undergone the insertion of a permanent pacemaker. Stimulation from the right ventricular apex in patients with a decreased left ventricular ejection fraction may increase mortality and worsen congestive heart failure, dyssynchrony caused by several mechanisms. Dyssynchrony may occur by increasing the delay between right and left ventricular contraction, worsening of ventricular remodeling, increasing the propensity of developing atrial fibrillation, and worsening of mitral insufficiency. Attempts at pacing from the interventricular septum or right ventricular outflow tract, to mitigate these changes, especially in patients with preserved left ventricular ejection fraction, may produce dyssynchrony similar to that observed with right ventricular apical stimulation [23]. Further studies are needed to fully assess this patient cohort.

At the present time, the decision to implant a CRT device is based on clinical and electrocardiographic data (wide QRS with an LBBB pattern) and not on echocardiographic criteria. Sporadic cases have described the benefit of CRT in patients with dyssynchrony and a narrow QRS, with improvement of LV function; however, this has not gained universal acceptance.

Despite the limited usefulness of echocardiographic techniques, an imaging technique (transthoracic echocardiography, three-dimensional echocardiography, or contrast angiography) has been described to guide the electrode location, assessing the asynchrony achieved with the active device [24]. Several data from classical transthoracic echocardiography may help to predict clinical improvement after the implantation of the resynchronization device: delayed septal and posterior wall contraction (≥130 ms) observed in M-mode and intraventricular dyssynchrony, defined as the difference between peak systolic contraction in contralateral walls >40 ms and a maximum delay >65 ms between anterior, inferior, septal, and basal lateral walls with tissue Doppler [25]. These methods have two problems: the low coincidence rate between observers (kappa index 0.1–0.39), and, as suggested in the PROSPECT study [21], no value was significantly associated with a higher clinical response.

Many studies define the relationship between a reduction in left ventricular end-systolic volume of at least 10% and a reduction in the width of the non-stimulated QRS (from 163 to 153 ms) and the stimulated QRS after implantation (from 146 to 121 ms) [26]. These data point at the same direction that those from other studies [27] and heighten the importance of placing the left ventricular electrode in the appropriate site and of properly programming the device, to achieve a narrow-paced QRS complex.

4. Optimization of resynchronization therapy

The problem of lack of response to resynchronization is complex. These devices would only be a priori indicated in the patients with greater probability of positive response. Patients with complete left bundle branch block and idiopathic dilated cardiomyopathy, with relative integrity of the His-Purkinje system, have a greater response than patients with left ventricular dysfunction of ischemic origin, with involvement of the conduction system by extensive areas of necrosis [28].

The absence of myocardial viability in the lateral region of the left ventricle, evaluated by magnetic resonance, makes more improbable positive response after cardiac resynchronization therapy, even though there are no echocardiographic data of asynchrony [29]. In addition, not every electrode implanted through the coronary sinus that stimulates the left ventricle has resynchronization capacity accompanied by clinical benefit.

The programming of the devices is important mainly in two parameters: the atrioventricular interval and the interventricular interval. It seems necessary to optimize the atrioventricular interval because an excessive elongation of the interval between atrial and ventricular systoles can lead to decreased cardiac output [30]. A direct observation of the transmitral flow pattern should be made by transthoracic echocardiography, attempting to separate the E and A waves and eliminate diastolic mitral regurgitation. Programming the interventricular interval sometimes produces nonsimultaneous biventricular pacing, which may be more effective than simultaneous pacing. It is more important to assess the echocardiographic response of the patient than the degree of QRS narrowing induced by therapy (which is a poor marker of clinical response to resynchronization). Interventricular delay can be measured by conventional pulsed Doppler and intraventricular asynchrony by the delay between peak septum and left ventricular posterior wall contraction in M-mode. It is not clear whether these intervals should be optimized in all patients and the order in which they should be done. But it should be emphasized that this optimization should not be done according to an algorithm, but individualized based on the response of each patient [30].

A survey carried out in Spain by the implantation centers of cardiac resynchronization devices [31] showed that the main obstacles for implantation are the difficulty in introducing the electrode in the selected vein (51%) and the poor electrode stability (26%). Seventy-three percent of centers do not perform any technique to optimize the point of stimulation prior to implantation. The clinical response rate is 74 ± 9%. For nonresponders, 15% of electrophysiologists replaced the electrode at a different point, 39% placed an electrode via the epicardial route with thoracotomy, 3.5% performed multifocal stimulation in the left ventricle, and about half (47.6%) admitted that it has no alternative to optimizing medical treatment.

The best position of the electrode has traditionally been a vein in the lateral and basal region of the coronary sinus, which is accompanied by an improvement in echocardiographic resynchronization parameters [32]. The initial objective of the electrophysiologists, years ago, was the implantation of the electrocatheter in those veins. In the present moment, this approach is overcome, because the areas of maximum electrical delay are not always areas of greater alteration of contractility. Several electrical parameters have been described during implantation that can predict reverse remodeling/favorable clinical response [33, 34], such as non-paced QRS intervals (151 versus 126 ms) and delayed right ventricle-left ventricle activation interval (93 versus 69 ms), greater in responders. One study [35] describes that the implantation of the electrocatheter in the right ventricle guided by the maximum electrical delay in the outflow tract, apex, or septum increases the response rate to the standard right ventricular apex implant.

Alternative stimulation points have been evaluated, which may be indicated in some patients where there may be inadequate functioning due to anatomical data, inadequate stimulation thresholds, electrode twisting or anchorage electrode, etc. The efficacy of left ventricular pacing from the lateral wall has been described [36]. Transeptal access may be useful in patients with difficulty in localizing the coronary sinus [37, 38], although it has the drawbacks of requiring long-term anticoagulation and the possibility of increasing mitral insufficiency [39]. Triangular stimulation can also be performed, with two electrodes implanted in the right ventricle (apex and outflow tract) and one in the left ventricle [40–42]. We can think about this pacing technique in patients in whom the left ventricular electrode cannot be placed endocardially, or in patients with heart failure, with extensive transmural myocardial scarring in posterior and lateral walls of the left ventricle, or even in patients with previous classic pacemaker with indication of upgrading/improvement of their performance. Although this technique seems to be less aggressive, its benefit appears smaller. Other authors [43, 44] use His-bundle pacing, which may be effective in patients with non-wide QRS, and may induce a greater QRS narrowing, although this is not always accompanied by an improvement in LV function. Few studies [45] describe Purkinje fiber pacing, which is similar to conventional pacing, and may be useful in patients with ischemic heart disease, with more stable stimulation in cases of myocardial damage.

Recent advances in design and materials of electrocatheters and guides have been accompanied by higher success rates in the implant [46]. The steerable positioning system of the catheter-guided catheter [47] achieves a nonsignificant improvement in the success rate of transvenous implant (93.7% versus 91.2% of the conventional method), with shorter implant time and less use of radiographic contrast. Easy maneuvers [48] may facilitate the progression of the electrocatheter through an unfavorable venous tree; with a second hydrophilic guide mounted in parallel with another one, the coronary sinus is accessed with a catheter of wide curvature, an angiography is done to assess the nature of the obstacle, and the first guide is inserted into the chosen vein to achieve the advance of the electrocatheter. Anatomical abnormalities such as the presence of a Thebesian valve, a fenestrated Thebesian valve, or an inadequate ratio of its size to the diameter of the ostium of the coronary sinus can be solved mostly with these two strategies [49].

A significant advance in this field is the quadripolar electrocatheter of the left ventricle [50]. Four electrodes are arranged along the 4.7 cm distal, allowing up to ten stimulation configurations, which means a greater probability of achieving an effective stimulation without the need to reposition the electrode. It has several advantages: adequated pacing thresholds, greater electrocatheter stability with low rates of electrode displacement, infrequent pacing of the phrenic nerve, pacing from basal left ventricle positions—apparently with better performance and ability to pacing around the scar tissue of the myocardium—and improved cardiac output in the medium to long term. Multipoint stimulation improves cardiac contractility to a greater extent than classical biventricular pacing [51], with an increase in the left ventricular ejection fraction of 12.7% compared to 6.7% in classic resynchronization [52].

Several intelligent resynchronization therapy algorithms have been recently developed. The algorithm called adaptive CRT pacing stimulates the left ventricle synchronously only when there is intrinsic activation of that ventricle, producing a fusion beat. This more physiological electrical programming gets different results [53, 54], so it cannot yet be widely recommended.

In the 80s and the early 90s, there was no routine optimization of the device after its implantation. Unlike in recent years, optimization of the therapy is performed a few weeks after implantation, using simple echocardiographic measurements, since the atrioventricular and interventricular intervals may be different in each individual and change over time. Several studies [55–57] show improved cardiac failure data and even improved survival in patients with scheduled post-implant visits. At these visits, problems can be detected with early correction and improvement of the prognosis of these patients (malignant ventricular arrhythmias, atrial fibrillation, ventricular pacing time of less than 90–95%, diaphragmatic pacing, inadequate electrode pacing, etc.). One work with methodological problems [58] found no such improvements with scheduled visits after the implant. It seems, therefore, that the option of frequent monitoring after the implant is better. The RESPOND CRT clinical trial (Clinicaltrials.gov: NCT01534234) is currently being conducted to evaluate the effectiveness of automatic optimization algorithms versus optimization based on echocardiographic criteria.

Remote monitoring is a technology that is increasingly used today and that may be more important in the future. The transmission of programmed and patients' response data is performed from a device implanted to the specialist's office [59]. It makes a closer follow-up in order to optimize the therapy and relieves the saturation of specialists' offices. The IN-TIME study [60] shows less worsening of cardiac failure data and nonsignificant mortality reduction in patients with implantable cardioverter defibrillator or mixed—resynchronization + defibrillator—devices. Recent clinical guidelines of the Spanish Society of Cardiology [4] recommend the implantation of devices with remote monitoring functionality (recommendation IIa, level of evidence A).

http://dx.doi.org/10.5772/64611

5. Treatment of resynchronization nonresponder patients

The evaluation of the patient who does not respond to resynchronization should be systematic (**Table 2**), taking into account the elements of the device, and cardiac and extracardiac patient data [61].

1.	To assess the ECG with and without pacemaker/resynchronization, arrhythmias
2.	To interrogate the device: sensing and capturing atrial and ventricular thresholds, atrioventricular and interventricular delays, physiological sensors
3.	To check the position of the electrodes: chest X-ray, fluoroscopy
4.	To verify the effect of resynchronization by echocardiography: Doppler parameters, mitral flow, dP/dt, intraventricular and interventricular dyssynchrony, atrioventricular and interventricular delay optimization
5.	To check for proper intake of basal medication
6.	To check for comorbidities

Table 2. Stepwise approach of the patient who does not respond to cardiac resynchronization.

It is desirable that biventricular stimulation be active about 100% of beats, even during exercise. The atrioventricular or interventricular intervals with echocardiographic control may be optimized, with pre-excitation of the left ventricle or simultaneous biventricular contraction. These changes may increase cardiac output in relation to the intrinsic cardiac rhythm and factory settings of the device.

The presence of atrial fibrillation leads to loss of left ventricular catheterization or to fusion/pseudofusion beats with ineffective resynchronization. Fusions or pseudofusions may not be detected by the device, so the percentage of stimulation may be falsely normal. This data should be exposed by reviewing the paths recorded in the device memory. If the sinus rhythm cannot be recovered, it is important to control the ventricular rate to ensure ventricular capture, sometimes even with an atrioventricular node ablation. The presence of frequent ventricular extrasystoles can inhibit pacing of the left ventricular lead and thus reduce the effectiveness of resynchronization; therefore, a percutaneous ablation can be considered.

Some nonresponder patients have loss of catheter capture. The beats produced by biventricular stimulation have a QRS axis in the upper right quadrant of the frontal plane and a dominant R wave in V1. If we observe a predominantly negative complex in V1 lead, we should suspect loss of capture or nonoptimal position of the left ventricular electrode, and its replacement can be considered.

The localization of the left ventricular lead may influence the response to resynchronization. Chest X-ray (posteroanterior and lateral projection images) and fluoroscopy are the methods of choice. The recommendation is to implant the electrode in a collateral branch of the coronary sinus (from basal to mediolateral or posterolateral) if there is an adequate vein to host the electrode.

The anterior position of the electrode is accompanied by a lack of response. And, the apical pacing can induce heterogeneous activation of the left ventricle. Electrocardiographic patterns of the left or right branch block, or intraventricular conduction disorder, can add greater variability in the activation pattern, so an implant should be performed by assessing the response in an individualized way.

In patients without positive clinical response to a left ventricular electrode in a nonoptimal position, the option of implanting a second electrode should be assessed. Computed tomography can be done to assess the anatomy of the branches of the coronary sinus. If the endocardial implant is not feasible, an epicardial approach via a mini-thoracotomy or a transeptal endocardial implant should be assessed. Before, an evaluation of the a priori morbidity of this new implant and the degree of compensation of other comorbidities of the patient should be made.

Despite the described limitations, it is mandatory to perform an echocardiography of the patient who does not improve with resynchronization. It is recommended to evaluate several aspects:

- The transmitral filling profile, which can improve acutely with the resynchronization. If the transmitral filling period is too short, less than 40–45% of the cycle duration, it can be optimized by prolonging atrioventricular delay. If the atrioventricular interval is too long, it may improve the resynchronization response by shortening that period. These data are not static and change over time, so it is suggested to optimize it preferably with echocardiography every 6 months.
- We can find data of favorable response to resynchronization, such as immediate reduction of functional mitral regurgitation, acute increase of left ventricular dP/dt (contractility index), and disappearance of the initial systolic inward movement of the interventricular septum [62].
- Another element of favorable response is the decrease in intraventricular dyssynchrony, measured as a decrease in the difference in the interval of aortic and pulmonary preeyection. In these cases an individual optimization of the interventricular interval is recommended. If there is no improvement, consider changing the position or the performance of the left ventricular electrode, or even cancel it/remove it.

One final aspect, but not less important, is the verification of compliance with the medication for treating heart failure. Up to 25% of patients without a resynchronization response do not take their prescribed medication [63].

There may be involuntary medication suppression, due to progressive renal insufficiency or adverse effects, with worsening of the condition. In addition, patients with arrhythmias may require antiarrhythmic treatment. The comorbidities of these patients (diabetes, ischemic heart disease, vascular and cerebral diseases) may attenuate the beneficial effects of resynchronization. Worsening renal function, anemia, and arterial hypotension are associated with poor prognosis in resynchronized patients. It has already been commented that the inverse remodeling is more pronounced in non-ischemic patients than in ischemic patients.

Optimizing the response to resynchronization, with that patient-focused individual approach (**Table 2**), can maximize the beneficial effect of cardiac resynchronization.

Author details

García García Miguel Ángel[1]*, Martínez Cornejo Alfonso[2] and Rosero Arenas María de los Ángeles[2]

*Address all correspondence to: mangelesymangel@hotmail.com

1 Intensive Care Unit, Hospital de Sagunto, Valencia, Spain

2 Center of Primary Care of Cheste, Valencia, Spain

References

[1] McMurray JJV, Petrie MC, Murdoch DR et al. Clinical epidemiology of heart failure: public and private health burden. Eur Heart J 1998; 19(suppl): 9–16.

[2] Cleland JG, Daubert JC, Erdmann E et al. The effect of cardiac resynchronization on morbidity and mortality in heart failure. N Engl J Med 2005; 352: 1539–1549.

[3] Yancy CW, Jessup M, Bozkurt B et al. 2013 ACCF/AHA guideline for the management of heart failure: executive summary: a report of the American College of Cardiology Foundation/American Heart Association Task Force on practice guidelines. Circulation 2013; 128: 1810–1852.

[4] Brignole M, Auricchio A, Baron-Esquivias G et al. 2013 Guidelines on cardiac pacing and cardiac resynchronization therapy. The task force on cardiac pacing and resynchronization therapy of the European Society of Cardiology (ESC). Eur Heart J 2013; 34: 2281–2329.

[5] Brambatti M, Guerra F, Matassini MV et al. Cardiac resynchronization therapy improves ejection fraction and cardiac remodelling regardless of patient's age. Europace 2013; 15: 704–710.

[6] Khatib M, Tolosana JM, Trucco E et al. EAARN score, a predictive score for mortality in patients receiving cardiac resynchronization therapy base on pre-implantation risk factors. Eur J Heart Fail 2014; 16: 802–809.

[7] Díaz-Infante E, Berruezo A, Mont Ll et al. Predictors of lack of clinical improvement at midterm follow-up with resynchronization therapy. Rev Esp Cardiol 2004; 57(4): 306–312.

[8] Al Hebaishi YS, Al Shehri HZ, Al Moghairi AM. Predictors of cardiac resynchronization therapy response: the pivotal role of electrocardiogram. Sci World J 2013, article ID 837086. http://dx.doi.org/10.1155/2013/837086

[9] Kang SH, Oh IY, Kang DY et al. Cardiac resynchronization therapy and QRS duration: systematic review, meta-analysis and meta-regression. J Korean Med Sci 2015; 30: 24–33.

[10] Coverstone E, Sheehy J, Kleiger R et al. The postimplantation electrocardiogram predicts clinical response to cardiac resynchronization therapy. PACE 2015; 38: 572–580.

[11] Sweeney MO, van Bommel RJ, Schalij MJ et al. Analysis of ventricular activation using surface electrocardiography to predict left ventricular reverse volumetric remodeling during cardiac resynchronization therapy. Circulation 2010; 121: 626–634.

[12] Kiani J, Agarwal SK, Kamireddy S et al. Relationship of electromechanical remodeling to survival rates after cardiac resynchronization therapy. Tex Heart Inst J 2013; 40: 268–273.

[13] Tereshchenko LG, Henrikson CA, Stempniewicz P et al. Antiarrhythmic effect of reverse electrical remodeling associated with cardiac resynchronization therapy. PACE 2011; 34: 357–364.

[14] Kogawa R, Nakai T, Ikeya Y et al. Dramatic response to cardiac resynchronization therapy with AV delay optimization in narrow QRS heart failure. Int Heart J 2015; 56(6): 671–675.

[15] Steffel J, Ruschitzka F. Superresponse to cardiac resynchronization therapy. Circulation 2014; 130: 87–90.

[16] Hsu JC, Solomon SD, Bourgoun M et al. Predictors of super-response to cardiac resynchronization therapy and associated improvement in clinical outcome. The MADIT-CRT study. JACC 2012; 59: 2366–2373.

[17] Imamura T, Kinugawa K, Nitta D et al. Complete left bundle branch block and smaller left atrium are predictors of response to cardiac resynchronization therapy in advanced heart failure. Circ J 2015; 79: 2414–2421.

[18] Duncan A, Wait D, Gibson D et al. Left ventricular remodeling and haemodynamic effects of multisite biventricular pacing in patients with left ventricular systolic dysfunction and activation disturbances in sinus rhythm: sub-study of the MUSTIC (Multisite Stimulation in Cardiomyopathies) trial. Eur Heart J 2003; 24: 430–441.

[19] García-Bolao I. Cardiac resynchronization therapy: when the pacing site really matters. Rev Esp Cardiol 2007; 60(2): 97–100.

[20] Turner MS, Bleasdale RA, Vinereanu D et al. Electrical and mechanical components of dyssynchrony in heart failure patients with normal QRS duration and left bundle branch block: impact of left and biventricular pacing. Circulation 2004; 109; 2544–2549.

[21] Chung ES, Leon AR, Tavazzi L et al. Results of the predictors of response to Cardiac Resynchronization Therapy (PROSPECT) trial. Circulation 2002; 40(9): 2608–2616.

[22] Marsan NA, Bleeker GB, Ypenburg C et al. Real-time three-dimensional echocardiography as a novel approach to assess left ventricular and left atrium reverse remodeling and to predict response to cardiac resynchronization therapy. Heart Rhythm 2008; 5(9): 1257–1264.

[23] Lange JM, Manzolillo H, Parras J et al. Right ventricular septal stimulation would produce similar bi-ventricular dyssynchrony as does apical stimulation in patients with normal ejection fraction. Arch Cardiol Mex 2014; 84(3): 183–190.

[24] Srivatsa SS. A proposed technique for right ventricular septal pacing. An article from the e-journal of the ESC Council for cardiology practice. Vol 12 No. 20–15 Apr 2014. https://

www.escardio.org/Journals/E-Journal-of-Cardiology-Practice/Volume-12/A-proposed-technique-for-right-ventricular-septal-pacing

[25] Zamorano J. Echocardiography and cardiac resynchronization therapy. Room for hope?. Rev Esp Cardiol 2008; 61(8): 800–802.

[26] Fernández-Pastor J, Cabrera-Bueno F, Linde-Estrella AL et al. Echocardiographic and electrical reverse remodeling in cardiac resynchronization therapy. Rev Esp Cardiol 2012; 65(6): 577–578.

[27] Molhoek SG, van Erven L, Bootsma M et al. QRS duration and shortening to predict clinical response to cardiac resynchronization therapy in patients with end-stage heart failure. Pacing Clin Electrophysiol 2004; 27: 308–313.

[28] Vasallo JA, Cassidy DM, Miller JM et al. Left ventricular endocardial activation during right ventricular pacing. Effect of underlying heart disease. J Am Coll Cardiol 1986; 7: 1228–1233.

[29] Bleeker GB, Kaandorp TA, Lamb HJ et al. Effect of posterolateral scar tissue on clinical and echocardiographic improvement after cardiac resynchronization therapy. Circulation 2006; 113: 969–976.

[30] Díaz-Infante E, Hernández-Madrid A, Brugada-Terradellas J et al. Consensus on cardiac resynchronization therapy. Rev Esp Cardiol 2005; 5(Suppl): 3B–11B.

[31] Hernández-Madrid A, Matía Francés R, Moro C et al. Cross-sectional Study of Cardiac Resynchronization Therapy in Spain. Indication, Implant Techniques, Optimization and Follow-Up. Rev Esp Cardiol 2012; 65(9): 826–834.

[32] Rosillo A, Verma A, Saad EB et al. Impact of coronary sinus lead position on biventricular pacing. Mortality and echocardiographic evaluation during long-term follow-up. J Cardiovasc Electrophysiol. 2004; 15: 1120–1125.

[33] Riva-Silva M, López-Gil M, Salgado-Aranda R et al. Value of intraoperative electrical parameters obtained during implantation of cardiac resynchronization therapy devices for the prediction of reverse remodeling. Rev Esp Cardiol 2014; 67(10): 855–857.

[34] Gold MR, Birgerdotter-Green U, Singh JP et al. The relationship between ventricular electrical delay and left ventricular remodeling with cardiac resynchronization therapy. Eur Heart J 2011; 32: 2516–2524.

[35] Miranda RJ, Nault M, Johri A et al. Maximal electric separation-guided placement of right ventricular lead improves responders in cardiac resynchronization defibrillation therapy. Circ Arrhythm Electrophysiol 2012; 5: 927–932.

[36] Derval N, Steendikj P, Gula LJ et al. Optimizing hemodynamics in heart failure patients by systemic screening of left ventricular pacing site. J Am Coll Cardiol 2010; 55: 566–575.

[37] Van Gelder BM, Bracke FA, Meijer A et al. Effect of optimizing the VV interval on left ventricular contractility in cardiac resynchronization therapy. Am J Cardiol 2004; 93: 1500–1503.

[38] Van Gelder BM, Scheffer MG, Meijer A et al. Transseptal endocardial left ventricular pacing: an alternative technique for coronary sinus lead placement in cardiac resynchronization therapy. Heart Rhythm 2007; 4: 454–460.

[39] Morgan J, et al. Alternate site cardiac resynchronization (ALSYNC): a prospective and multicentre study of left ventricular endocardial pacing for cardiac resynchronization therapy. Eur Heart J 2016; 37: 2118–2127.

[40] Yoshida K, Seo Y, Yamasaki H et al. Effect of triangle ventricular pacing on hemodynamics and dyssynchrony in patients with advanced heart failure: a comparison study with conventional bi-ventricular pacing therapy. Eur Heart J 2007; 28: 2610–2619.

[41] Bazan V, Delclos J, Vallès E et al. Estimulación bifocal ventricular derecha. "Una alternativa en la terapia de resincronización cardiaca". Cuadernos de estimulación cardiaca 2011; 4(11): 11–15. http://secardiologia.es/images/stories/secciones/estimulacion/cuadernos-estimulacion/11/estimulacion-bifocal-en-vd.pdf

[42] Yoshida K, Yokohama Y, Seo Y et al. Triangle ventricular pacing in a non-responder to conventional bi-ventricular pacing. Europace 2008; 10: 502–504.

[43] Sashida Y, Mori F, Arashi H et al. Improvement of left ventricular function by permanent direct His-bundle pacing in case with dilated cardiomyopathy. J Arrhythm 2006; 22: 245–250.

[44] Padeletti L, Lieberman R, Schreuder J et al. Acute effects of His bundle pacing versus left ventricular and right ventricular pacing on left ventricular function. Am J Cardiol 2007; 100: 1556–1560.

[45] Hamaoka M, Mine T, Kodani T et al. Hemodynamic effects of Purkinje potential pacing in the left ventricular endocardium in patients with advanced heart failure. J Arrhythm 2015; 31: 371–375.

[46] Alonso C, Leclercq C, d'Allonnes FR et al. Six years experience of transvenous left ventricular lead implantation for permanent biventricular pacing in patients with advanced heart failure: technical aspects. Heart 2001; 86: 405–410.

[47] Er F, Yüksel D, Hellmich M et al. Comparison of conventional versus steerable-catheter guided coronary sinus lead positioning in patients undergoing cardiac resynchronization device implantation. PLoS One 2015; 10(11): e0143292. doi:10.1371/journal.pone.0143292

[48] Arbelo E, Medina A, Bolaños J et al. Double-wire technique for implanting a left ventricular venous lead in patients with complicated coronary venous anatomy. Rev Esp Cardiol 2007; 60: 110–117.

[49] Arbelo Lainez E, Medina Fernández-Aceytuno A, Bolaños J et al. The Thebesian valve as determinant of the difficulty of access to the coronary sinus: anatomical and angiographic observations. Rev Esp Cardiol 2004; 57(Suppl 2): 145.

[50] D'Ortencio A, Bevacqua RJ. Results of patients with resynchronization therapy using a quadrupole electrode in the left ventricle. Insuf Card 2013; 8(3): 142–148.

[51] Thibault B, Dubuc M, Khairy P et al. Acute haemodynamic comparison of multisite and biventricular pacing with quadripolar left ventricular lead. Europace 2013; 15: 984–1067.

[52] Alonso P, Andrés A, Osca J et al. Improvement in hemodynamics and contractility with multipoint left ventricular pacing in cardiac resynchronization therapy. Rev Esp Cardiol 2014; 67 (10): 859–61.

[53] Birnie D, Lemke B, Aonuma K et al. Clinical outcomes with synchronized left ventricular pacing: analysis of the adaptative CRT trial. Heart Rhythm 2013; 10: 1368–74.

[54] Thibault B, Ducharme A, Harel F et al. Evaluation of resynchronization therapy for heart failure I. (GREATER_EARTH). Left ventricular versus simultaneous biventricular pacing in patients with heart failure and a QRS complex >=120 ms. Circulations 2011; 124: 2874–81.

[55] Hess PL, Mi X, Curtis LH et al. Follow-up of patients with new cardiovascular implantable electronic devices: is adherence to the experts' recommendations associated with improved outcomes?. Heart Rhythm 2013; 10(8): 1127–1133.

[56] Urbanek B, Chudzik M, Klimczak A et al. Whether noninvasive optimization of AV and VV delays improves the response to cardiac resynchronization therapy. Cardiol J 2013; 20 (4): 411–417.

[57] Delnoy PP, Ritter P, Naegele H et al. Association between frequent cardiac resynchronization therapy optimization and long-term clinical response: a post hoc analysis of the clinical evaluation on advanced resynchronization (CLEAR) pilot study. Europace 2013; 15: 1174–1181.

[58] Ellenbogen KA, Gold MR, Meyer TE et al. Primary results from the SmartDelay determined AV optimization: a comparison to other AV delay methods used in cardiac resynchronization therapy (SMART-AV) trial: a randomized trial comparing empirical, echocardiography-guided, and algorithmic atrioventricular delay programming in cardiac resynchronization therapy. Circulation 2010; 122: 2660–2668.

[59] García Urra F, Porres Aracama JM. Telemonitoring: actual state 2015. http://www.impulsorevista.es/monitorizacion-remota-estado-actual/

[60] Hindricks G, Taborsky M, Glikson M et al. Implant-based multiparameter telemonitoring of patients with heart failure (IN-TIME): a randomized controlled trial. Lancet 2014; 384 (9943): 583–590.

[61] Kutyifa V, Breithardt OA. How to assess the nonresponder to cardiac resynchronization therapy—a comprehensive stepwise approach. Rev Esp Cardiol 2012; 65(6): 504–510.

[62] Kedia N, Ng K, Apperson-Hansen C et al. Usefulness of atrioventricular delay optimization using Doppler assessment in mitral inflow in patients undergoing cardiac resynchronization therapy. Am J Cardiol 2006; 98: 780–785.

[63] Mullens W, Grimm RA, Verga T et al. Insights from a cardiac resynchronization optimization clinic as part of a heart failure disease management program. JACC 2009; 53: 765–773.

Chapter 5

Utility of Cardiac Implantable Electronic Devices in Patients with Chagas Disease and Systolic Heart Failure

Guillermo Mora

Additional information is available at the end of the chapter

http://dx.doi.org/10.5772/67079

Abstract

Chagas disease (CD) is the principal cause of congestive heart failure (CHF) in areas where the disease is endemic and migration has increased the likelihood of these diseases being the probable cause of CHF in other countries of the world. Sudden cardiac death (SCD) is the most common cause of death in CD (55–65%). Implantable cardioverter defibrillator (ICD) is useful in the secondary prevention of SCD, but there is less information regarding primary prevention. The evidence supporting the use of cardiac resynchronization therapy (CRT) in CHF of chagasic etiology is poor; however, one should apply current guidelines regarding the insertion of these devices in patients with Chagas disease and CHF.

Keywords: Chagas disease, congestive heart failure, sudden cardiac death, implantable cardioverter defibrillator, cardiac resynchronization therapy

1. Introduction

Chagas disease (CD), also known as American trypanosomiasis, was discovered by Carlos Chagas in 1909, is caused by infection with the protozoa *Trypanosoma cruzi* (*T. cruzi*). CD had become widely recognized by the World Health Organization as a neglected tropical disease [1]. *T. cruzi* may be transmitted through blood transfusion, organ transplantation, congenital transmission, or ingestion of contaminated food [2, 3]. However, *T. cruzi* infection most often occurs via vectorial transmission by a type of reduviid bug called a triatomine. *T. cruzi* is excreted in the feces of an infected triatomine bug onto human skin or near mucous membranes. The parasites breach the dermis through excoriations in the skin and gain systemic access [4]. Inoculation is followed by an incubation period of 1 to 2 weeks; it is characterized by parasitemia and subsequent immune response; and 10–30% of infected individuals will begin to exhibit nonspecific symptoms of acute CD, including abdominal pain, anorexia, fever, lymphadenopathy, rash, malaise and localized swelling around the site of infection [5]. However, the majority of individuals become asymptomatic carriers of *T. cruzi* or indeterminate phase.

Approximately one-third of patients progress to the determinate phase in which cardiac symptoms and signs arise from progressive myofibril fibrosis and conduction system injury [6]. This phase begins after several decades during which there are no clinically overt symptoms of organ damage or abnormal electrocardiographic results; 30–40% of asymptomatic carriers will develop chronic CD characterized by dilated cardiomyopathy leading to congestive heart failure (CHF) and/or by development of gastrointestinal disorders [7].

The Pan American Health Organization (PAHO) estimates between 8 and 12 million people seropositive [8]. Annual deaths are of less variable, ranging from 10,600 to 12,500 [9]. In Latin American countries, 100 million people are at risk of infection and 300,000 new cases are reported each year [10].

The United States (US) Centers for Disease Control and Prevention have reported more than 300,000 immigrants living in the US infected with *T. cruzi* [11]. In 2010 CD was responsible for 550,000 (274,000–1,069,000) disability-adjusted life years (DALYs), a measure that captures both premature mortality and nonfatal health loss [12].

The diagnosis of chronic CD should be suspected in patients from endemic areas (Central and South America) with dilated cardiomyopathy or electrocardiographic abnormalities like right bundle-branch block associated or not with left anterior hemiblock (LAHB). Definitive diagnosis is based on serology to detect immunoglobulin G antibodies to *T. cruzi*, using at least two serological tests of different principles. The most commonly used are enzyme-linked immunosorbent assay (ELISA), indirect immunofluorescence (IIF) and indirect hemagglutination (IHA).

2. Sudden cardiac death and Chagas disease

Sudden cardiac death (SCD) is the most common cause of death in CD (55–65%), followed by congestive heart failure (CHF) (25–30%) and cerebral or pulmonary embolism (10–15%) [13]. Although SCD may affect asymptomatic patients, it affects patients with evidence of chronic heart disease, particularly those with CHF in the majority of cases [14]. The prevalence of SCD in CD patients with CHF is about 46% [15], whereas in a general unselected CD population is 29% [16]. The prevalence also changes in different areas, varying from 29% in non-endemic to 37% in endemic areas [16, 17]. Most SCD cases are in patients with manifest chagasic cardiomyopathy and mainly between 30 and 50 years of age, being rare after the sixth decade of life [14]. On the other hand, up to 20% of patients who die suddenly do not report previous symptoms [14]. SCD may exceptionally occur as a result of rupturing of the left ventricular apical aneurysm, massive cardioembolic stroke, or pulmonary embolism [18, 19]. However, in the overwhelming majority of cases, it is essentially an arrhythmic phenomenon.

In a study of ten chagasic patients who died suddenly with an ambulatory Holter, bradyarrhythmias were the final event in one patient. Ventricular fibrillation (VF) was the final arrhythmia in nine patients; torsades de pointes was the precursor in six and sustained ventricular tachycardia (VT) in three patients [20]. From the studies carried out in Chagas' disease patients receiving implantable cardioverter defibrillator (ICD) therapy, it has become clear that sustained VT is the most frequently observed life-threatening ventricular arrhythmia, although in about 30% of patients who develop VF without having sustained TV as a precursor [21].

The mechanism underlying the tachyarrhythmia episodes in Chagas' disease patients is micro-reentry. There is impressive reparative confluent fibrosis intermingled with normal myocardium. In addition, there is also a diffuse mononuclear cell infiltrate. The association of these two myocardial abnormalities can provoke the appearance of multiple areas of slow conduction in the vicinity of scars, forming foci of reentry disseminated throughout the heart, mainly in the epicardial areas [22, 23]. Another point that deserves further consideration is the autonomic dysfunction; studies in patients with chronic CD have clearly demonstrated parasympathetic derangement in patients with chronic CD [24]. In a study of 52 patients with Chagas cardiomyopathy with pacemaker or ICD, we found more positive serological response against 2e-m2MAChR (antibody that recognizes the muscarinic acetyl choline receptor type II) than in patients with pacemaker or ICD without CD (32.7 vs 3.8% $p < 0.01$) [25].

The risk of SCD is not similar for every patient. Rassi et al. [26] developed and validated a risk score for predicting death in 424 patients followed for a mean of 7.9 years. They identified six independent prognostic factors: New York Heart Association (NYHA) class III or IV (5 points), cardiomegaly on chest radiography (5 points), segmental or global wall motion abnormality on echocardiogram (3 points), non-sustained VT on Holter monitoring (3 points), low QRS voltage (2 points) and male sex (2 points). This score classifies in three groups of risk for 10 years mortality: low risk (0–6 points, 10%), intermediate risk (7–11 points, 44%) and high risk (12–20 points, 84%). In this study the rate of SCD was 2.4% for a year. Although the score risk was development for total mortality, all of the variables were also strong predictors for SCD, except low QRS voltage.

Other risk factors include syncope, spontaneous sustained VT, abnormalities on the 12-lead electrocardiogram or echocardiogram, or sustained TV induced by programmed ventricular stimulation (PVS). In 28 chagasic patients with sustained TV over a mean follow-up of 3816 months, deaths occurred in 13 patients (46.4%) and resulted from SCD in seven subjects [27]. Interestingly, in this study the prognosis was similar with non-sustained VT. The presence on echocardiogram of left ventricular dilatation and left apical ventricular aneurysm was associated with SCD [15]. In the same way, the presence of Q waves, frequent premature ventricular contractions, left anterior fascicular block (LAFB), or QT interval dispersion has been established predictors of SCD [28]. In 78 patients with CD and non-sustained VT, PVS was carried out and sustained monomorphic VT was induced in 25 patients (32%) and VF in four (5.1%). Induction of sustained ventricular arrhythmias was the independent and main variable that predicted cardiac death (OR 2.17 CI 95% 1.23–3.83) [29].

In summary CD is associated with SCD, most commonly through VF, often preceded by sustained VT. There is a higher risk group that may be established by clinical criteria and invasive or noninvasive procedures (**Table 1**).

• Syncope
• NYHA class III–IV
• Male sex
• Spontaneous sustained VT
• Q wave
• Left anterior fascicular block
• QT interval dispersion
• Non-sustained VT
• Frequent premature ventricular contractions
• Cardiomegaly on chest radiography
• Left ventricular dilatation
• Left apical ventricular aneurysm
• Segmental motion abnormality
• Sustained VT induced with PVS
NYHA, New York Heart Association; VT, ventricular tachycardia; PVS, programmed ventricular stimulation.

Table 1. Risk factors associated with sudden cardiac death in chagasic patients.

3. ICD in Chagas disease

3.1. Secondary prevention of SCD

The use of ICD has become a main therapeutic strategy for prevention of sudden death.

A meta-analysis of AVID (Antiarrhythmics versus implantable defibrillators), CIDS (Canadian Implantable Defibrillator Study) and CASH (Cardiac Arrest Study Hamburg) that evaluated utility of ICD in secondary prevention of SCD demonstrated that ICD therapy was associated with 50% (p = 0.0001) reduction in arrhythmic mortality and a 28% (p = 0.006) reduction in total mortality [30]. Today, ICD is considered class I A recommendation in patients recovered of SCD [31]. However, in these studies there is no information about chagasic patients.

In a study of secondary prevention, 65 chagasic patients were compared with 70 non-chagasic patients and were followed for the median time of 266 days. Appropriate ICD therapy occurred in 32 (49.2%) chagasic patients and in 19 (27.1%) of the control group (p = 0.005). There was a statistically significant difference in event-free survival in the Chagas group. Finally, CD doubles the risk of the patient to have appropriate therapy (HR = 2.2) and appropriate therapy or death (HR 2.2). The annual mortality rate was 17% [32].

Some authors have proposed the use of amiodarone alone for secondary prevention in chagasic patients. The limited evidence available does not favor this hypothesis. A study compared the outcomes of Chagas' heart disease patients with life-threatening ventricular arrhythmias, who were treated with ICD with a historical group treated with amiodarone alone. The ICD group (76 patients) had higher use of beta-blocker ($p < 0.0001$). Amiodarone was also used in 90% of the ICD group. Therapy with ICD plus amiodarone produced 72% reduced risk of all-cause mortality ($p = 0.007$) and a 95% reduced risk of sudden death ($p = 0.007$) compared with amiodarone-only therapy. The follow-up was 36 ± 16 months for the ICD group and 35 ± 17 months for the control group. There are ten deaths (4.7% per year) in the ICD group and nine deaths (11% per year) in the control group [33].

Several studies have evaluated over a long-term follow-up period the efficacy of ICD. A study included 116 consecutive patients with CD and an ICD implanted for secondary prevention. The average follow-up was 45 months. In this survey 58 (50%) patients had appropriate shocks. A total of 31 patients died (7.1% annual mortality rate) [34]. Another study assessed a cohort with 65 patients (51 in secondary prevention) with median follow-up of 40 ± 26.8 months. Among the patients 23 (36.5%) had appropriate shocks. A total of 13 (20%) patients died (6.1% of annual mortality rate) and there was no sudden death [35]. A survey with 90 patients with ICD for secondary prevention found, with median follow-up of 756 ± 581 days, 31 (34%) deaths (16.4% of annual mortality rate) [36]. Maybe the largest study in secondary prevention with chagasic patients evaluated 148 subjects with mean follow-up was 12 ± 7 months. During the follow-up 15 patients died (10.2%) [37].

Patients with chronic CD with life-threatening ventricular arrhythmias have an annual mortality rate between 8.6% and 11% when they are treated with amiodarone [33, 38]. However, survival probability at 3 years of follow-up is 30% in patients with no treatment and 20% treated with quinidine or procainamide [39].

No randomized clinical trial has assessed the effect of ICD therapy on outcome of Chagas' disease patients with malignant ventricular arrhythmias thus far. However, with available information it is obvious that patients without treatment (mortality 70% at 3 years) or with class IA antiarrhythmic (mortality 80% at 3 years, possibly due to antiarrhythmics) have high mortality [39] and need other options. Amiodarone has been used for a long term in these patients, with an annual mortality rate between 8.6 and 11% [33, 38].

ICD is associated with an annual mortality rate between 6.1 and 17% [32–37]. Thus, the impact of ICD implantation on all-cause mortality has shown inhomogeneous results, possibly related to differences among populations and treatments in the studies. The only study that compared ICD plus amiodarone against amiodarone alone demonstrated reduction of the risk of all-cause mortality and sudden death. Patients with left ventricular ejection fraction (LVEF) < 40% derived more survival benefit [33].

Although some authors have suggested the need of a randomized clinical trial to demonstrate the usefulness of ICD in this population [40], most groups working with chagasic patients are extrapolating the secondary prevention ICD indications proposed by international guidelines [31] as reflected by the I Latin American guidelines for the diagnosis and treatment of Chagas heart disease [41].

On the other hand, these patients have differences with other patients with non-Chagas cardiomyopathy. In the meta-analysis of the ICD secondary prevention trials, the authors found that the mean LVEF was 34 ± 15% [30]. Conversely, the mean LVEF among the studies with chagasic patients is higher (37–47%); it is suggesting that CD is more arrhythmogenic heart disease or less dependent of the ventricular damage [32–37]. Moreover, a substantial number of the included patients had no left ventricular dysfunction.

Another difference between chagasic or non-chagasic patients with ICD for secondary prevention is the age at the time of implantation. In the meta-analysis was 63 ± 11 years, while in chagasic patients was lower (54–59 years) [32–37].

There are differences with life-threatening ventricular arrhythmias; Chagas' disease patients tend to experience more shocks. In a study during the first 6 months of follow-up, 17 of the 20 (85%) chagasic patients received at least one appropriate therapy. In the control group (ischemic patients), 18 of the 35 (51%) received one ICD shock (RR 1.6; $p < 0.02$) [42]. In other studies, the frequency of appropriate shock was 36–64% in the follow-up for 1–2 years [32–37].

Otherwise, several groups have shown predictors of all-cause mortality in patients with Chagas heart disease receiving ICD. The most common predictors of mortality were NYHA class III (HR 3.09 95% CI 1.37-6.98, p = 0.0064), LVEF (HR 0.97 95% CI 0.94-0.99, p = 0.04) and low cumulative right ventricular pacing < 40% (HR 0.23 95% CI 0.11-0.49, p = 0.0001) [34].

In another study the only predictor was the number of shocks; probability of survival for patients receiving more than four shocks by day 30 post-implant was 75% at 30 days and 19% at 60 days, whereas probability of survival for patients receiving up to four shocks by day 30 were 97% at 30 days, 96% at 120 days, 94% at 270 days and 89% at at 360 days of follow-up (p = 0.00005). Mean life expectancy was 2.1 months (95% CI 0.79–3.4) in patients receiving more than four shocks by day 30 and 46.5 months in patients receiving up to four shocks by day 30 (p = 0.0005) [36]. Pereira et al. found predictors of poor prognosis: a LVEF < 30% and low education [35] and another group showed that patients older than 65 years of age and LVEF < 30% were independent predictors of all-cause 1 year mortality [37]. It is important to note that in the studies of secondary prevention, the medical treatment was incomplete for the use of beta-blocker, angiotensin-converting enzyme inhibitors (ACEI)/Angiotensin II receptor blockers (ARB) or spironolactone.

Although several authors have suggested that amiodarone is the initial management in chagasic patients with VT without hemodynamic instability and ICD in other patients [43], most

Secondary prevention of SCD
• ICD therapy + amiodarone (class I)
Primary prevention of SCD
• ICD therapy in chagasic patients with LVEF < 40% (class I)
Treatment of CHF
• CRT in patients with LVEF < 35% + OMT + LBBB + NYHA class II–IV (class I)
• CRT in patients with LVEF < 35% + OMT + RBBB + NYHA class III–IV (class II B)

SCD, sudden cardiac death; ICD, implantable cardioverter defibrillator; LVEF, left ventricular ejection fraction; OMT, optimal medical treatment; LBBB, left bundle branch block; NYHA, New York Heart Association; RBBB, right bundle branch block.

Table 2. Indications of ICD and CRT in chagasic patients.

groups recommend ICD therapy as an initial approach possibly associated with the use of amiodarone (**Table 2**) [31].

3.2. Primary prevention of SCD

If the evidence, in the management of patients with life-threatening ventricular arrhythmias, is not of great quality, the information is even poor in primary prevention of SCD. As expected, no randomized controlled study has been carried out.

In the only study available, Cardinalli-Neto et al. included 32 patients with a LVEF < 35%, receiving standard therapy for chronic systolic heart failure and to have a reasonable expectation of 1-year survival after device implantation; all patients were on NYHA class II and none had syncope. Nineteen (59%) patients had a positive serology for CD. Notably, 87% of patients were on beta-blocker and 100% were on ACEI/ARB.

Sustained VT was detected in four (21%) patients with Chagas heart disease and in two (15%) patients with non-Chagas (p = NS). VF was observed in four (21%) patients with Chagas cardiomyopathy and in two (15%) with non-Chagas patients (p = NS). Median time to first event was 78 (34–151) days in Chagas and 173 (71–593) days in non-Chagas patients (p = 0.005). Median follow-up was 292 (78–845) days in Chagas and 654 (159–987) days in non-Chagas (p = 0.005) here was no difference in mortality) [44].

Non-sustained VT is an independent predictor of all-cause mortality and SCD in patients with Chagas cardiomyopathy with LVEF from 30 to 50% [45]. In these patients the prognosis role of PVS has been studied. In 78 chagasic patients with mean LVEF 48% and non-sustained VT, electrophysiologic testing was realized. In 25 (32%) out of 78 patients, sustained VT was induced. During a mean follow-up of 56 ± 38 months, 22 (28%) patients died, SCD affecting 16 (73%) of them. A significant association between inducible sustained VT and SCD was found ($p < 0.05$). All patients induced with sustained VT received amiodarone [29].

Actually, European guidelines recommend using ICD in chagasic patients with LVEF < 40% [31]. However, a significant number of SCD occur in patients with LVEF > 40% and in these subjects, there is no adequate way to establish their risk. PVS might be an option, but new and larger studies are necessary (**Table 2**).

4. Heart failure in Chagas disease

After the acute phase of the disease, most patients enter a clinically asymptomatic chronic phase without electrocardiographic or radiological abnormalities in the heart, which has been described as the indeterminate chronic form. Nevertheless, when these individuals are subjected to echocardiogram or radionuclide, ventriculography is common to find abnormalities; endomyocardial biopsy shows abnormalities in 60% of the cases [46]. Every year 2.5% would evolve into cardiac or digestive symptomatic forms [47]. CHF affects approximately 5% of a general unselected CD population and up to 76% of patients followed at outpatient services in tertiary referral centers [48].

Chagasic cardiomyopathy is a chronic myocarditis that affects all chambers, the parasympathetic cardiac nerves and all levels of the system [49]. Four possible mechanisms have been suggested: cardiac parasympathetic neuronal depopulation, immune-mediated myocardial injury, parasite persistence in cardiac tissue with secondary antigenic stimulation and coronary microvascular abnormalities [25, 49].

CD is the principal cause of CHF in areas where the disease is endemic [50]. Mortality is still high even in the current era of heart failure therapy (around 20% annual) [51]. When compared with other etiologies, outcome is poorer [52].

CD is associated with ventricular conduction delay. In a large population date base on primary case patients, 7590 had CD. The electrocardiogram showed right bundle branch block (RBBB) in 22.7%, left anterior hemiblock (LAHB) in 22.5%, RBBB + LAH in 13,74% and left bundle branch block (LBBB) in 3.07% of patients [53]. In chagasic patients an increase in QRS duration correlated with a decrease in LVEF and increase in left ventricular diastolic diameter [54]. On echocardiographic evaluation, the presence of apical or inferobasal aneurysms in the left ventricle is common (**Figures 1** and **2**).

The beneficial effects on survival and morbidities of drugs observed in non-Chagas disease heart failure are extrapolated to Chagas' disease patients. Medical treatment of CD heart failure is not supported by strong evidence. Small studies have shown that neurohormonal inhibition can improve both symptoms and left ventricular function. However, a systematic review of Cochrane found very low-quality evidence for the effects of carvedilol compared with placebo for treating heart failure in people with CD [55]. On the other hand, chagasic

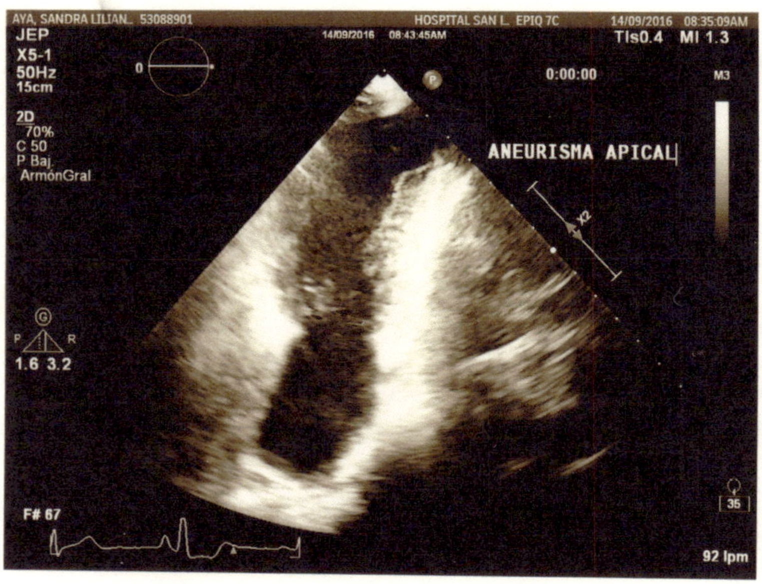

Figure 1. Echocardiogram with apical aneurysm in the left ventricle in a patient with Chagas cardiomyopathy.

http://dx.doi.org/10.5772/67079

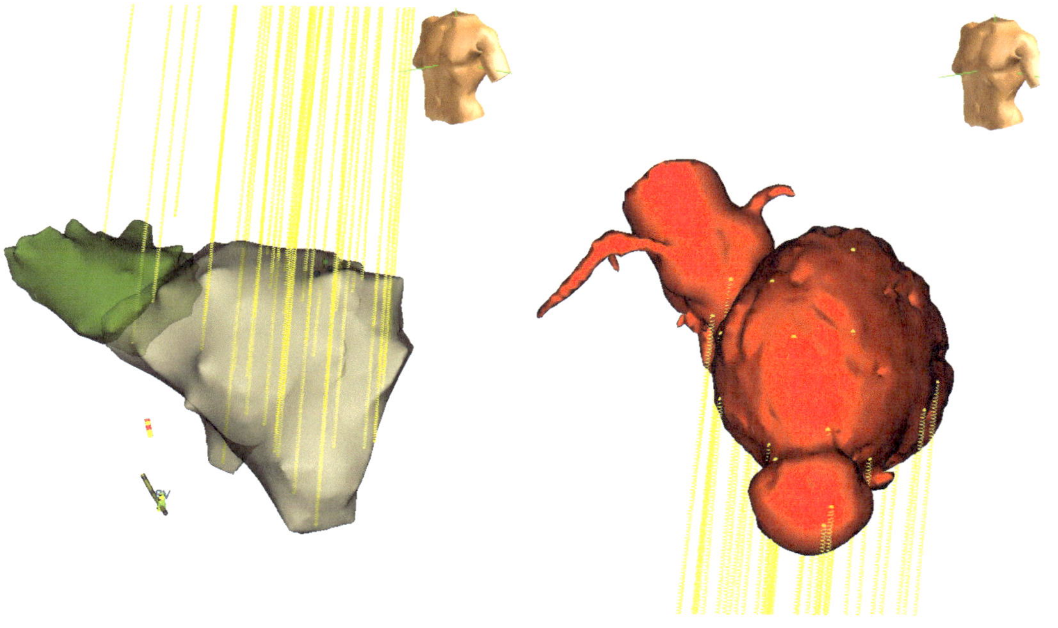

Figure 2. Real-time image integration of the left ventricle with computed tomography and electroanatomical map with EnSite NavX. Image of the left ventricle with apical and inferobasal aneurysm.

patients frequently have lower blood pressure and a higher incidence of bradyarrhythmias and may not tolerate target doses of angiotensin-converting enzyme inhibitors (ACEI) and beta-blockers.

In conclusion CHF secondary to CD has higher mortality and problems with the neurohormonal blockade, related to difficulty in reaching optimum doses of beta-blockers and ACEI.

5. Cardiac resynchronization therapy

Cardiac resynchronization therapy (CRT) is an established therapeutic modality for patients with non-Chagas heart disease with LVEF < 35%, in appropriate medical management and LBBB with a QRS 150 mseg (class I). In patients with non-LBBB pattern, the recommendation is class II [56].

Evidence of the usefulness of CRT in CD is scarce. Araujo et al. analyzed 72 chagasic patients in NYHA class III or IV, who underwent CRT. The average clinical follow-up was 46.6 month (4–79). At the end of the evaluation, 87.4% of patients were in NYHA class I or II and they had increase of the LVEF. There was an overall mortality of 34.7% of the patients underwent implantation of the electrode of the left ventricle through a left anterior mini-thoracotomy. All patients were on beta-blocker therapy and 70% on ACEI. Mean QRS duration was 148.1 17 mseg, 47% was with LBBB, 15% on permanent right ventricular paging and mean LVEF was 27.3 ± 7.7% [57].

In another study 30 chagasic patients in NYHA class III or IV undergone to right ventricular bifocal pacing. No change in the LVEF after 6 months of follow-up. However, a marked increase in arrhythmic episodes was observed.. The mortality rate was 43% in the first year of follow-up.

In a small study, 29 patients (52% chagasic) with conventional pacemakers implanted in the right ventricular apical area, in NYHA class III/IV refractory to drug therapy and LVEF < 35%, underwent CRT. During the follow-up of 22.7 ± 13 months, 86.2% of the patients benefited from CRT. However, there was no differential analysis of the chagasic patients [58].

There is low frequency of complete LBBB (16%) in chagasic patients with CHF. The most frequently found intraventricular conduction dysfunction is RBBB alone or with LAFB [51]. Nowadays, there is controversial evidence to support the use of CRT in patients without LBBB. Recently, a small study with 78 patients with RBBB showed that single-site pacing of the right ventricular septum near the proximal right bundle resulted in a marked decrease in QRS duration and often normalized the ECG [59], so that there may be new alternatives of stimulation in this patient group.

In conclusion the evidence of CRT in CHF of chagasic etiology is poor; however, in patients with LBBB, LVEF < 35% with adequate medical therapy CRT is indicated. In patients with RBBB, CRT is probably unhelpful. If RBBB is attached to LAFB, some authors consider useful biventricular pacing, but studies proving this theory are necessary.

6. Other treatments

Heart transplantation is an option in patients with refractory CHF. There are many concerns with regard to the usefulness in chagasic patients because of *T. cruzi* infection reactivation, the adequate immunossuppresive protocol and long-term results. A systematic review found that survival probability at 1 month, 1 year, 4 years and 10 years of follow-up was 83, 71, 57 and 46%, respectively. Such an outcome was better than that seen in non-Chagas patients [60]. Later, a study with 107 chagasic patients with follow-up between 30 and 168 months found the highest mortality (42.9%) [61]. Transplantation in Chagas' disease has several problems that differ from other etiologies due to the possibility of disease reactivation and the increased possibility of emergence of cancers. However, transplantation is the only treatment able to modify the natural progression of the disease in its terminal phase.

The utility of the left ventricular circulatory support as bridge to heart transplantation has been little studied. A study with 6 patients with chagasic cardiomyopathy, the mean time of circulatory support was 27 days, authors found that 2 patients were bridged to heart transplantation successfully and other four patients died.

Sustained VT is common in chagasic patients. The most frequent mechanism is scar-related reentry; the circuit may be subepicardial, intramyocardial, or subendocardial (**Figure 3**). Reports have described a higher prevalence of epicardial VT (37%). The electrophysiological signs show delayed potentials predominantly in the target area during mapping in sinus

http://dx.doi.org/10.5772/67079

rhythm and presystolic activity. Meso-diastolic and continuous activities are also frequent in the original place of VT. The critical isthmus of the reentrant circuit may be confirmed by entrainment maneuvers or interruption of VT during the application of RF in these places. In general, the site of origin of well-tolerated recurring VT can be identified and the VT interrupted in 60–80% of the patients, but rapid and poorly tolerated SVT is frequently induced in the final assessment of the procedure. During long-term follow-up, at least 50% of the patients have clinical relapse [41]. The main indication for catheter ablation is ICD shocks despite antiarrhythmic therapy.

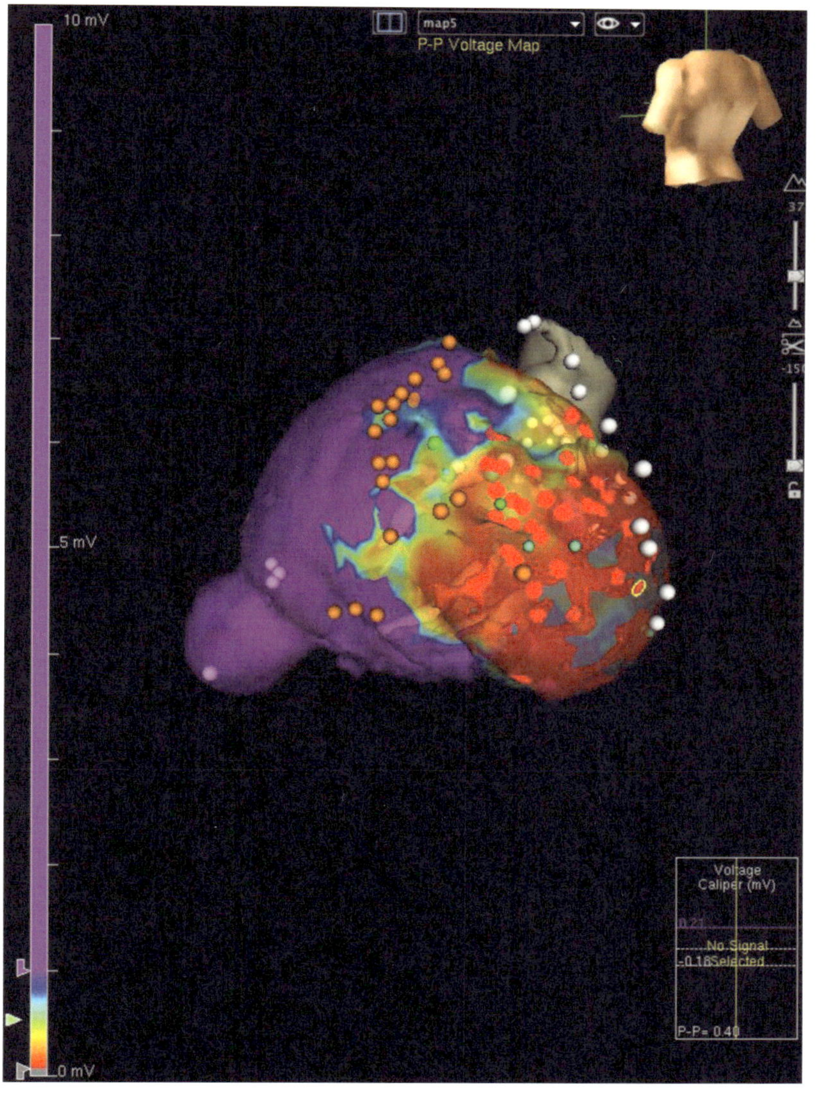

Figure 3. Image of **Figure 2** with voltage sinus rhythm map showing extensive scar inferobasal.

7. Conclusions

CD is an important cause of CHF in Latin America; migration has become this disease in a probable cause of CHF in other countries of the world. CD is associated with high prevalence of SCD; ICD is indicated as therapy class I in secondary prevention of SCD. ICD is also indicated as therapy class I in primary prevention of SCD in chagasic patients with LVEF < 40% with optimal medical treatment (OMT). The utility of PVS should be investigated in patients with non-sustained VT and LVEF > 40%.

CHF is very common in patients with CD. CRT is indicated as therapy class I in patients with LBBB + LVEF < 35% + OMT. Indication in patients with non-LBBB is controversial and new and large studies are necessary.

Author details

Guillermo Mora

Address all correspondence to: gmorap@unal.edu.co

Universidad Nacional de Colombia, Hospital Universitario Nacional, Bogotá, Colombia

References

[1] Bonney K. Chagas disease in the 21st century: a public health success or an emerging threat? Parasite 2014; 21: 1–10.

[2] Teixeira AR, et al. Chagas disease. Postgrad Med J 2006; 82: 788–98.

[3] Howard EJ, et al. Frequency of the congenital transmission of *Trypanosoma Cruzi*: a systematic review and meta-analysis. BJOE 2014; 121: 22–33.

[4] Rossi M, Ramos S, Bestetti R. Chagas' heart disease: clinical pathological correlation. Front Biosci 2003; 8: e94–109.

[5] Tanowitz HB, et al. Chagas' disease. Clin Microbiol Rev 1992; 5: 400–19.

[6] Rossi M. Patterns of myocardial fibrosis in idiopathic cardiomyopathies and chronic chagasic cardiopathy. Can J Cardiol 1991; 7: 287–94.

[7] Rassi A Jr., Rassi A, Marin-Neto JA. Chagas disease. Lancet 2010; 375: 1388–402.

[8] OPS/WHO/NTD/ID. Quantitative estimate of Chagas disease in the Americas. OPS/HDM/CD/425-06. Washington DC: Organización Panamericana de la Salud; 2006.

[9] GBD 2013. Mortality and causes of death collaborators. Global, regional and national age-sex specific all-cause and cause-specific mortality for 240 causes of death, 1990–2013

http://dx.doi.org/10.5772/67079

a systematic analysis for the Global Burden of Disease Study 2013. Lancet 2015; 385: 117–71.

[10] World Health Organization. World Health Assembly report. Geneva (Switzerland): World Health Organization; 2010: 1–4.

[11] Bern C; Montgomery SP. An estimate of the burden of Chagas disease in the United States. Clin Infect Dis 2009; 49: e52–4.

[12] Murray CJ, et al. Disability-adjusted life years (DALYs) for 291 diseases and injuries in 21 regions, 1990 2010: a systematic analysis for the Global Burden of Disease Study 2010. Lancet 2012; 380: 2197–223.

[13] Rassi A Jr., et al. Sudden death in Chagas' disease: review. Arq Bras Cardiol 2009; 76: 75–96.

[14] Bestetti RB, et al. Clinical and morphological characteristics associated with sudden cardiac death in patients with Chagas' disease. Eur Heart J 1993; 14: 1610–4.

[15] Bestetti RB, et al. Predictors of sudden cardiac death for patients with Chagas' disease: a hospital-derived cohort study. Cardiology 1996; 87: 481–7.

[16] Manzullo EC, Chuit R. Risk of death due to chronic chagasic cardiopathy. Mem Inst Oswaldo Cruz 1999; 94 (Suppl. 1): 317–20.

[17] Lopez ER, et al. Contribution to the study of the pathological anatomy of chagasic hearts suddenly died. Rev Soc Bras Med Trop 1975; 9: 269–81.

[18] Oliveira JSM, Barbieri-Neto J. Chagas cardiomyopathy. "Broken aneurysm of the tip". Arq Bras Cardiol 1970; 23: 335–8.

[19] Carod-Artal FJ, et al. Chagasic cardiomyopathy is independently associated with ischemic stroke in Chagas' disease. Stroke 2005; 36: 965–70.

[20] Mendoza I, Moleiro F, Marques J. Sudden death of Chagas disease. Arq Bras Cardiol 1992; 59: 3–4.

[21] Cardinalli-Neto A, Greco OT, Bestetti RB. Automatic implantable cardioverter-defibrillators in Chagas' heart disease patients with malignant ventricular arrhythmias. Pacing Clin Electrophysiol 2006; 29: 467–70.

[22] Bestetti RB, Cardinalli-Neto A. Sudden Cardiac death in Chagas' heart disease in the contemporary era. Int J Cardiol 2008; 131: 9–17.

[23] Henz BD, et al. Simultaneous epicardial and endocardial substrate mapping and radiofrequency catheter ablation as first-line treatment for ventricular tachycardia and frequent ICD shocks in chronic chagasic cardiomyopathy. J Interv Card Electrophysiol 2009; 26: 195–205.

[24] Oliveira JSM. A natural human model of intrinsic heart nervous system denervation: Chagas cardiopathy. Am Heart J 1985; 110: 1092–8.

[25] Tovar NC, Echeverry MC, Mora G. Presence of antibodies to cardiac neuroreceptors to muscarinic acetyl choline receptor type II (anti-m2MAChR). in patients with Chagas disease and pacemakers. Biomédica 2009; 29: 476–84.

[26] Rassi A Jr., et al. Development and validation of a risk score for predicting death in Chagas' heart disease. N Eng J Med 2006; 355: 799–808.

[27] Sarabanda AV, Martin-Neto JA. Predictors of mortality in patients with Chagas' cardiomyopathy and ventricular tachycardia not treated with implantable cardioverter-defibrillators. Pacing Clin Electrophysiol 2011; 34: 54–62.

[28] Salles G, et al. Prognostic value of QT interval parameters for mortality risk stratification in Chagas' disease. Circulation 2003; 108: 305–12.

[29] Silvia RM, et al. Predictive value of clinical and electrophysiological variables in patients with chronic chagasic cardiomyopathy and nonsustained ventricular tachycardia. Arq Bras Cardiol 2000; 75: 33–47.

[30] Connolly SJ, et al. Meta-analysis of the implantable cardioverter defibrillator secondary prevention trials. Eur Heart J 2000; 21: 2071–8.

[31] Priori S, et al. 2015 ESC Guidelines for the management of patients with ventricular arrhythmias and the prevention of sudden cardiac death. Eur Heart J 2015; 36: 2793–867.

[32] Barbosa MP, et al. Efficacy and safety of implantable cardioverter-defibrillators in patients with Chagas disease. Europace 2013; 15: 957–62.

[33] Gali WL, et al. Implantable cardioverter-defibrillators for treatment of sustained ventricular arrhythmias in patients with Chagas' heart disease: comparison with a control group treated with amiodarone alone. Europace 2014; 16: 674–80.

[34] Martinelli M, et al. Long-term follow-up implantable cardioverter-defibrillator for secondary prevention in Chagas' heart disease. Am J Cardiol 2012; 110: 1040–5.

[35] Pereira FT, et al. Long term follow-up of patients with chronic Chagas disease and implantable cardioverter-defibrillator. Pacing Clin Electrophysiol 2014; 37: 751–6.

[36] Cardinalli-Neto A, et al. Predictors of all-cause mortality for patients with chronic Chagas' heart disease receiving implantable cardioverter defibrillator therapy. J Cardiovasc Electrophysiol 2007; 18: 1236–40.

[37] Di Toro D, et al. Predictors of all-cause 1-year mortality in implantable cardioverter defibrillator patients with chronic Chagas' cardiomyopathy. Pacing Clin Electrophysiol 2011; 34: 1063–9.

[38] Leite LR, et al. The impact of syncope during clinical presentation of sustained ventricular tachycardia on total and cardiac mortality in patients with chronic chagasic heart disease. Arq Bras Cardiol 2001; 77: 446–52.

http://dx.doi.org/10.5772/67079

[39] Rassi Jr A, et al. Ventricular arrhythmias in Chagas' disease. Diagnostic, prognostic and therapeutic features. Arq Bras Cardiol 1995; 65: 377–87.

[40] Rassi A Jr. Implantable cardioverter-defibrillators in patients with Chagas heart disease: misperceptions, many questions and the urgent need for a randomized clinical trial. J Cardiovasc Electrophysiol 2007; 18: 1241–3.

[41] Andrade JP, et al. I Latin American guidelines for the diagnosis and treatment of Chagas heart disease: executive summary. Arq Bras Cardiol 2011; 96: 434–42.

[42] Rabinovich R, et al. Time to first shock in implantable cardioverter defibrillator (ICD) patients with Chagas cardiomyopathy. Pacing Clin Electrophysiol 1999; 22: 202–5.

[43] Bestetti R, Cardinalli-Neto A. Device therapy in Chagas disease heart failure. Expert Rev Cardiovasc Ther 2012; 10: 1307–17.

[44] Cardinalli-Neto, et al. Implantable cardioverter-defibrillator therapy for primary prevention of sudden cardiac death in patients with severe Chagas cardiomyopathy. Int J Cardiol 2011; 150: 94–5.

[45] Carrasco HA, et al. Prognostic implications of clinical, electrocardiographic and hemodynamic findings in chronic Chagas' disease. Int J Cardiol 1994; 43: 27–38.

[46] Pereira-Barreto AC, et al. Right ventricular endomyocardial biopsy in undetermined form of Chagas disease. Am Heart J, 1986; 111: 307–12.

[47] Dias JC, et al. The indeterminate form of human chronic Chagas disease. A clinical and epidemiological review. Rev Soc Bras Med Trop 1989; 22: 147–56.

[48] Bestetti RB et al. Treatment of chronic systolic heart failure secondary to Chagas heart disease in the current era of heart failure therapy. Am Heart J 2008; 156: 422–30.

[49] Martin-Neto JA, et al. Pathogenesis of chronic Chagas heart disease. Circulation 2007; 115: 1109–23.

[50] Bertolino ND, et al. Prognostic impact of Chagas disease in patients awaiting heart transplantation. J Heart Lung Transplant 2010; 29: 449–53.

[51] Theodoropoulos TA, et al. Predictors of all-cause mortality in chronic Chagas heart disease in the current era of heart failure therapy. Int J Cardiol 2008; 128: 22–9.

[52] Barbosa AP, et al. Comparison of outcome between Chagas cardiomyopathic and idiopathic dilated cardiomyopathy. Arq Bras Cardiol 2011; 97: 517–25.

[53] Marcolino A, et al. Electrocardiogram and Chagas disease: a large population database of primary care patients. Glob Heart 2015; 10: 167–72.

[54] Nacimento BR, et al. The prognostic significance of electrocardiographic changes in Chagas disease. J Electrocardiol 2012; 45: 43–8.

[55] Marti-Carvajal AJ, Kwong JS. Pharmacological interventions for treating heart failure in patients with Chagas cardiomyopathy. Cochrane Datebase Syst Rev 2016; 7: CD009077.

[56] Yancy CW, et al. 2013 ACCF/AHA guideline for the management of heart failure: a report of the American College of Cardiology Foundation/American Heart Association task force on practice guidelines. Circulation 2013; 128: 240–327.

[57] Araujo EF, et al. Cardiac resynchronization therapy in patients with chronic Chagas cardiomyopathy: long-term follow up. Rev Bras Cir Cardiovasc 2014; 29: 31–6.

[58] Silva RT, et al. Functional behavior of patients with conventional pacemakers undergoing cardiac resynchronization. Arq Bras Cardiol 2008; 90: 138–43.

[59] Giudici MC, et al. Right ventricular septal pacing in patients with right bundle branch block. J Electrocardiol 2015; 48: 626–9.

[60] Bestetti RB, Theodoropoulos TA. A systematic review of studies on heart transplantation for patients with end-stage Chagas' heart disease. J Card Fail 2009; 15: 249–55.

[61] Fiorelli AI, et al. Heart transplantation in 107 cases of Chagas' disease. Transplant Proc 2011; 43: 220–4.

Section 3

Role of Trans-Catheter Ablation in Patients with Systolic Heart Failure

Chapter 6

Transcatheter Ablation of Atrial Fibrillation in Patients with Chronic Heart Failure

Antonio Di Monaco, Federico Quadrini,
Nicola Vitulano and Massimo Grimaldi

Additional information is available at the end of the chapter

http://dx.doi.org/10.5772/67024

Abstract

Atrial fibrillation (AF) is the most frequent of all cardiac arrhythmias and it is associated with an increased risk of stroke, systemic embolism and heart failure. Patients with AF have a twofold increased risk of death and fivefold increased risk of stroke compared with those without AF. In patients with heart failure (HF), AF ablation improves left ventricular (LV) function over short- and long-term follow-ups, especially compared with medical treatment. Furthermore, AF ablation in HF patients relates to a significant improvement in quality of life, functional class and exercise tolerance, possibly related to the improvement in LV function and hemodynamic status of the patients. Finally, data showed that restoration of sinus rhythm in this setting of patients reduced the incidence of stroke and death. In this review, we reported all the major data regarding atrial fibrillation therapy in patients with heart failure.

Keywords: atrial fibrillation ablation, heart failure, quality of life, left ventricular function, atrial fibrosis

1. Incidence and pathogenesis of atrial fibrillation in heart failure

Atrial fibrillation (AF) is defined as a cardiac arrhythmia characterized by the surface ECG showing 'absolutely' irregular RR intervals and absence of distinct P waves. Irregular atrial electrical activity, represented by the "f" waves, may be seen in some ECG leads, most often in lead V1, the "f-f" interval is variable and usually shorter than 200 ms [1]. An irregular pulse should always raise the suspicion of AF, but an ECG recording is necessary to diagnose AF [1].

From a clinical point of view, AF can be categorized into five subtypes based on the presentation and duration of the arrhythmia: (1) patient who presents with AF for the first time; (2) paroxysmal AF is self-terminating, usually within 48 h, but it may continue for up to 7 days; (3) persistent AF is present when an AF episode either lasts longer than 7 days or requires termination by cardioversion; (4) AF is considered as long-standing persistent when the arrhythmia has lasted for ≥1 year; (5) permanent AF, when the presence of the arrhythmia is accepted by the patient (and physician) and when it is decided to adopt a rate control strategy [1] (**Figure 1**).

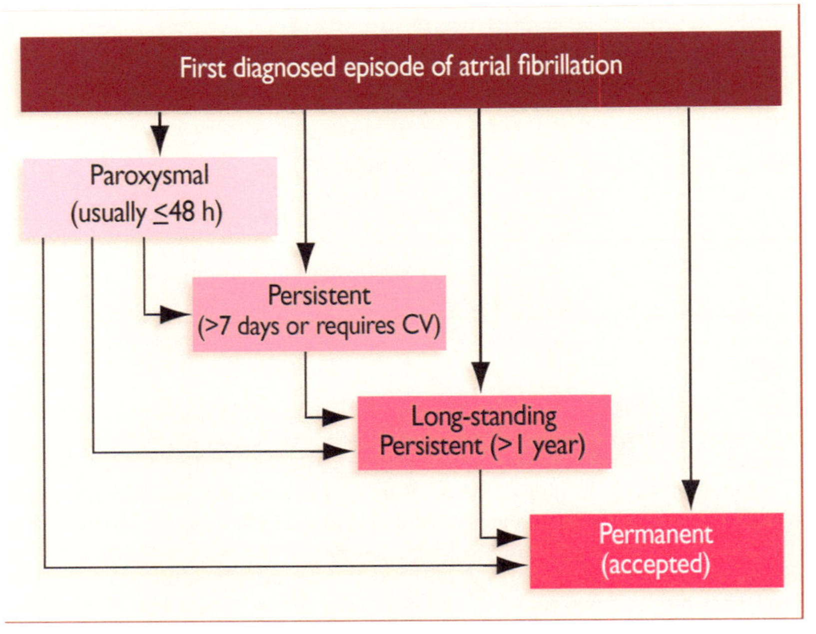

Figure 1. European Society of Cardiology guidelines for classification of atrial fibrillation [1].

Atrial fibrillation, the most frequent of all cardiac arrhythmias, is associated with an increased risk of stroke, systemic embolism (SE) and heart failure (HF). Patients with AF have a twofold increased risk of death and fivefold increased risk of stroke compared with those without AF [1–6].

Atrial fibrillation has multiple adverse clinical implications. The loss of atrial systole and the irregular, fast heart rate contribute to symptoms such as palpitations and reduced exercise tolerance and also predispose to the development of intracardiac thrombus and systemic thromboembolism. Atrial fibrillation can also cause tachycardia-mediated cardiomyopathy or worsening of preexisting heart failure [3].

Whereas anticoagulation treatment reduced the risk for stroke, large randomized trials failed to demonstrate any significant mortality benefit of a pharmacologically based rhythm control strategy even in patients with left ventricular dysfunction when compared with a rate control strategy [7–11].

This has led to a widespread belief that restoration of sinus rhythm (SR) does not improve prognosis. However, in-depth analysis of these trials demonstrated that the restoration of SR was associated with a 47% lower risk for death compared with continuing AF.

Besides having a good safety profile, catheter ablation therapy for AF has proved effective in establishing and maintaining SR. Induction of AF requires an initiating trigger and perpetuation occurs because triggering activity is sustained or because of the presence of a susceptible atrial substrate. Premature atrial ectopy has been shown to be the most frequent trigger for AF. Observations in patients with dual-chamber pacemakers revealed that 48% of AF episodes were triggered by premature atrial beats, 33% were preceded by bradycardia and 17% were sudden in onset [12]. Also, continuous cardiac monitoring in postoperative patients demonstrated that supraventricular premature beats induced AF in 72–100% of cases [13].

Endocardial mapping revealed that the origin of ectopic activity initiating AF is located inside the pulmonary veins (PV) in 89–94% of cases and that AF is most often triggered by repetitive focal PV discharges [14–18].

Catheter ablation targeting the fascicles, which connect the PVs to the left atrium, leads to electrical isolation of the PVs. Interestingly, after electrical isolation, up to 58% of PVs display slow, dissociated activity and some sustain ongoing tachycardia dissociated from the left atrium in SR, emphasizing the arrhythmogenic potential of these structures [19, 20].

Indeed, besides being triggers for AF, PVs can also be responsible for the perpetuation of AF. In a small series of patients who had irregular focal discharges initiating and perpetuating AF, foci at the ostium of PVs were found to be the drivers of sustained AF in 66%. Focal radiofrequency (RF) delivery targeting these foci eliminated AF in all these patients [21].

In addition, a spatial gradient in cycle length, with the PVs activating at a higher frequency than the nearest atrial tissue, has been found in some patients and this reinforces the role of PVs as AF perpetuators [22–25].

The involvement of the PVs in the maintenance of AF was further emphasized by the observation that PV isolation in paroxysmal AF led to a progressive increase in the AF cycle length, culminating in the termination of AF in 75% of patients. PV isolation rendered AF noninducible in 57% of patients and prevented relapse in 74% of patients [26]. These findings led to the venous wave hypothesis, postulating a role for PVs in maintenance of AF in most patients with paroxysmal AF [27]. Later, spectral analysis and dominant frequency mapping revealed that the dominant frequency and the highest dominant frequency were spatially distributed near the PVs in most of patients with paroxysmal AF [28]. Put together, these observations emphatically substantiate the role of PVs in the initiation and maintenance of nonpermanent forms of AF.

Although elimination of PV arrhythmogenicity has been highly effective for paroxysmal AF, it has modest efficacy for persistent AF suggesting that mechanisms beyond the PVs also contribute to perpetuation of AF in these patients. A number of ablation strategies have been proposed: linear ablation, ablation of complex fractionated atrial electrograms, ablation of intrinsic cardiac autonomics and ablation of rotors. Frequently these approaches are performed in combination, to target these substrate-related mechanisms beyond the PV arrhythmogenicity, particularly in patients with persistent AF [1].

In the setting of heart failure, the increased filling pressure of atrial and ventricle contributes to the electroanatomic disarrangement of the muscle fibers providing a substrate for reentry and imparts electrical heterogeneity and arrhythmogenicity to onset AF. Histological examinations of atrial tissue in patients with AF show patchy fibrosis, which may contribute to the nonhomogeneity of conduction. Atrial biopsies from patients undergone to cardiac surgery show increase in cell size, loss of sarcoplasmic reticulum and atrial myofibrils, changes in mitochondrial shape, accumulation of glycogen granules, alteration in connexin expression and increase in extracellular matrix [1]. A multicenter trial has demonstrated that atrial fibrosis, as estimated by magnetic resonance imaging (MRI), is independently associated with the likelihood of recurrent AF and in particular an extensive fibrosis caused a low success rate after catheter ablation [29]. Furthermore, recent studies showed that transmural conduction is the predominant mechanism of breakthrough during atrial fibrillation demonstrating the substrate complexity of this arrhythmia [30].

Heart failure increases the risk of AF, with the mechanism of the arrhythmia being multifactorial. Furthermore, AF is an independent risk factor for the development of heart failure and both conditions frequently coexist. Atrial fibrillation in patients with heart failure predisposes to episodes of worsening heart failure and increases the risk of thromboembolic events [1]. Hospitalizations due to AF account for one-third of all admissions for cardiac arrhythmias. Acute coronary syndrome, aggravation of heart failure, thromboembolic complications and acute arrhythmia management are the main causes. In 30% of patients with AF, it is possible to find HF with NYHA II-IV and at the same time, in 30–40% of heart failure patients, AF is found. Heart failure can be both a consequence of AF (e.g., tachycardiomyopathy or decompensation in acute onset AF) and a cause of the arrhythmia due to increased atrial pressure and volume overload, secondary valvular dysfunction, or chronic neurohumoral stimulation.

In the past decade, it showed an increase of the incidence of AF, above all in patients with HF. Many factors have contributed to these epidemiological changes; first of all, the new therapeutic approach to the cardiovascular disease and the following growing average age of patients. A recent comparison between two survey showed a significant increase in the incidence of AF in patients with HF between 38.4% in 2005 and 50.4% in 2013 [31]. Marked unexplained interregional variations in the occurrence of stroke and mortality suggest that factors other than clinical variables might be important [31]. Prevention of death from heart failure should be a major priority in the treatment of atrial fibrillation.

2. Pharmacological treatment of atrial fibrillation in heart failure

2.1. Rhythm control vs. rate control

The optimal resting ventricular rate in patients with AF and HF could be between 60 and 100 bpm [32–34]. Van Gelder et al. [35] suggested that a resting ventricular rate of up to 110 bpm might still be acceptable and 2016 ESC AF guidelines recommend this threshold as the target for rate control therapy [33, 36–40], but a lower rate for patients with HF may be preferable (60–100 bpm). The optimal ventricular rate during exercise is also uncertain, but may be 110 bpm during light exercise [34].

Sinus rhythm, theoretically, offers physiological rate control, normal atrial activation and contraction, a normal sequence of atrioventricular (AV) conduction and AV valvular function and a regular rhythm.

Most clinical trials (PIAF, STAF, RACE, HOT CAFÉ, CABANA and AFFIRM) [1, 9–11, 41, 42] have reported no clear superiority of rhythm control. Furthermore, Crijns have reported that patients with AF and HF are unlikely to remain in sinus rhythm in the long-term and 2012 focus updated of ESC guidelines of the management of atrial fibrillation, that rhythm control should not be vigorously pursued in this clinical setting [1].

However, a subgroup analysis of AFFIRM reported that rhythm control may be useful in patients with left ventricular dysfunction. In this study, patients with depressed left ventricular function benefited significantly from rhythm control compared to rate control. The presence of sinus rhythm was associated with a lower risk of death [43].

2.2. Practical approach to rate control

Rate control in AF is based mainly on pharmacological depression of conduction through the AV node. In the presence of HF, this requires careful dose titration and can result in symptomatic bradycardia requiring permanent pacing. Beta-blockers are the preferred drugs in combination with digoxin (adjunctive therapy), because they provide optimal rate control at rest and during exercise in this setting of patients [1]. The AFFIRM study showed during long-term follow-up that beta-blockers achieved optimal rate control in 58% of patients [44]. In a subgroup analysis, patients with a history of HF and left ventricular ejection fraction <40%, successful rate control was observed with beta-blocker, with or without digoxin in 81% and with digoxin alone in 54%, at 1-year follow-up.

Atrioventricular (AV) nodal ablation may be the treatment of choice in the presence of symptoms intolerable to higher rates, despite the use of rate slowing agents. Investigators compared pharmacological rate control vs. AV node ablation in 66 patients with CHF and AF [45]. In this randomized study, both treatment arms were associated with alleviation of symptoms and an increase in functional capacity. Patients treated with the "ablate and pace" strategy had fewer symptoms with no changes in cardiac performance and quality of life. This strategy was not associated with a reduction of mortality.

2.3. Practical approach to rhythm control

The potential of amiodarone to maintain sinus rhythm in patients with AF and HF has been repeatedly shown in observational and prospective randomized controlled studies.

In CTAF study, therapy with amiodarone reduced the incidence of recurrent AF by 57% when compared with sotalol and propafenone [46]. In the CHF-STAT study, patients treated with amiodarone, converted to sinus rhythm more frequently (31.3% vs. 7.7% on placebo) compared to placebo, experienced fewer recurrences of AF and were less likely to develop new AF [47]. Amiodarone is a drug of choice for the management of AF associated with HF. In addition to its antiarrhythmic effects, it is useful in controlling ventricular rate response during recurrences [47].

Dronedarone is a drug similar to amiodarone, though is devoid of iodine with a theoretically safer adverse effect profile [1]. In the dronedarone atrial fibrillation study after electrical cardioversion (DAFNE) trial, dronedarone prolonged the mean interval to recurrence of AF by 55% compared with placebo, resulting in the spontaneous conversion to sinus rhythm in high percentage of patients. The results of the European trial in atrial fibrillation or flutter patients receiving dronedarone for the maintenance of sinus rhythm (EURIDIS) and American-Australian-African equivalent ADONIS showed that dronedarone was superior to placebo in the prevention of recurrent AF and effective in controlling the ventricular rate in over 1200 patients. However, the dronedarone in moderate to severe HF evaluating morbidity decrease (ANDROMEDA) study was stopped prematurely, as an interim safety analysis suggested an excess risk of death in patients on active treatment.

3. Ablation of atrial fibrillation in HF patients

Rhythm control with antiarrhythmic drugs has not been shown to confer benefit in randomized trials, neither in patients with HF nor in those without HF [7, 8]. The lack of benefits of antiarrhythmic drugs might reflect their poor (<50%) efficacy in maintaining sinus rhythm [8]. Conversely, ablative treatment in these patients can be highly effective in reducing morbidity and improving quality of life and functional capacity [7–9, 41–52]. However, patients with AF and left ventricular ejection fraction have more recurrences after a single procedure, thus requiring more repeat procedures, which increase costs and risks [53]. Recent studies [54–60] have demonstrated that nonpulmonary vein foci firing from the atrial chambers or other thoracic veins play an important role in initiating and maintaining AF in 3.2–62% of patients, depending on age, sex and comorbidities. Patients with HF usually have a more complex and diseased atrial substrate harboring more nonpulmonary vein foci, which could be responsible for the observed recurrence of AF or atrial tachyarrhythmia AT after pulmonary vein antrum isolation.

In a recent study, Zhao et al. [61] demonstrated that patients with left ventricular ejection fraction more often presented nonpulmonary vein triggers than in patients with normal ejection fraction; in patients with the long-term procedural outcome of pulmonary vein isolation ablation alone remain unsatisfactory with a 32.2% single-procedure success rate, whereas pulmonary vein isolation plus nonpulmonary vein triggers ablation significantly increases the success rate to 75.0%, which is comparable with the success rate of pulmonary vein isolation alone in patients with normal ejection fraction (75.0% vs. 81.7%).

Patients with low ejection fraction and paroxysmal atrial fibrillation had a higher prevalence of nonpulmonary vein triggers than patients with normal ejection fraction (69.1% vs. 26.6%). Many investigators [54–60] have addressed the importance of nonpulmonary vein triggers

http://dx.doi.org/10.5772/67024

for atrial fibrillation initiation and the reported incidence of nonpulmonary vein triggers in paroxysmal atrial fibrillation.

The basis for extensive left atrial ablation lies in the pathophysiology of atrial fibrillation itself [62]: atrial fibrillation perpetuating in a left atrium with significant substrate modifications and advanced structural and electrical remodeling has historically been targeted by linear lesions [63]. However, linear lesions and CFAE ablation may increase the risk of iatrogenic atypical atrial re-entries (flutter) or atrial tachycardias if not transmural, incomplete, or not perfectly anchored to electrically inert structures, counterbalancing the benefit derived by extensive atrial substrate modification [64].

Among the studies reporting AF ablation in patients with HF, 55% of the patients underwent PV isolation alone, with a large heterogeneity among studies (6–89%). None of the observational studies were designed to compare the efficacy of different AF ablation approaches. However, in the meta-analysis by Anselmino et al. [65] including the largest available population, there was no difference in AF ablation outcome, performing PV isolation alone when compared with additional linear ablation. Moreover, no data compared the different techniques to perform AF ablation (radiofrequency, cryoablation, laser, rotors and surgery) in patients with HF. Finally, recent data reported a higher success rate after AF ablation with a hybrid approach (percutaneous and surgical), but no data were published regarding patients with HF [1].

Larger randomized studies are needed to understand the optimal procedural protocol to adopt in patient with HF and symptomatic AF.

3.1. Paroxysmal vs. persistent atrial fibrillation ablation in heart failure

Several studies have suggested that catheter ablation of AF in the context of HF is relatively safe reporting that the complication rate was not different from that in patients with structurally normal hearts [7, 48–53, 65–85]. The success rate for catheter ablation of paroxysmal AF was similar in HF patients compared with non-HF patients (70–80%), whereas the success rate for persistent AF was markedly worse. In randomized studies, the success rate following a single procedure has been reported at 38–68%, rising to 50–88% after repeated procedures (2 or 3) at 6–12 months [52, 79–81]. Ullah et al [84] published an international multicenter registry from seven centers for patients with HF undergoing AF ablation (**Figure 2**). In this study with 1273 patients (171 with HF and 1102 without HF) and a median follow up of 3.1 years, the final procedure success rate was no different from paroxysmal AF (78.7% vs. 85.7%, $p = 0.186$), but significantly different for persistent AF (57.3% vs. 75.8%, $p < 0001$).

However, despite a lower success rate in patients with HF ablated for persistent AF, Zhu et al. [85] published a meta-analysis of three randomized controlled trials showing a significant improvement of LVEF (6.22%) and reduction of NYHA class and Minnesota living with heart failure questionnaires scores in patients with HF ablated for persistent AF compared with the medical rate control.

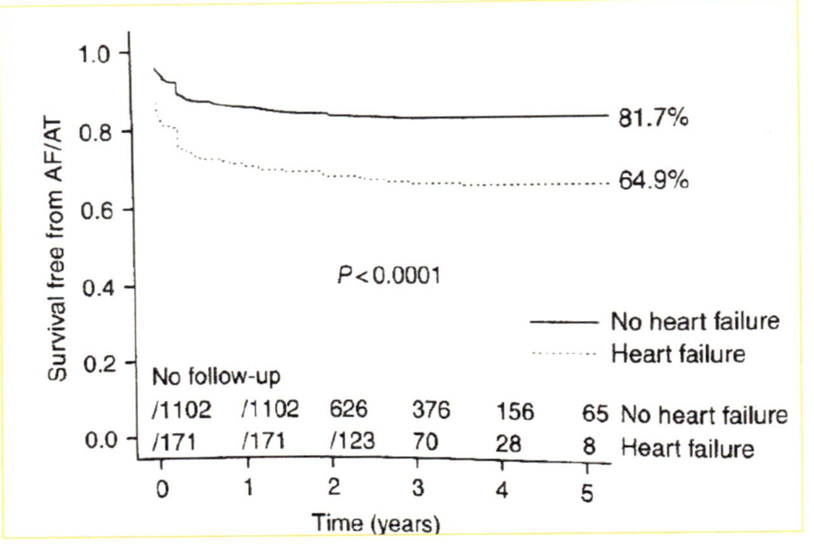

Figure 2. Freedom from atrial fibrillation and atrial flutter after ablation in patients with and without heart failure [84].

The lower success rate for catheter ablation for persistent AF in the HF group is likely multifactorial. Both HF and the conditions leading to HF increase the left atrial pressure and wall stress that causes progressive mitral regurgitation, which further impacts on left atrial pressure and remodeling. The result of these factors is more scarred and remodeled atria, which are more inclined to support AF.

3.2. Improvement in left ventricular function and heart failure

3.2.1. Symptoms after atrial fibrillation ablation

Atrial fibrillation ablations have been shown to improve the LV function during short- and long-term follow-up, when compared to medical therapy. Several meta-analyses regarding the usefulness of AF ablation in HF patients have been published [53, 65, 82, 83, 85]. In the first two works, including maximum 800 patients, the authors concluded that single AF ablation procedure in HF patients is less effective in patients without structural disease, but improves including redo procedures, obtaining a significant improvement in LV ejection fraction over follow-up [53, 82]. The third multicenter, collaborative meta-analysis, including more than 1800 patients [65], reported over a mean follow-up of 2 years a significant improvement in LV ejection fraction and a reduction in the proportion of patients with severely depressed LV function. This finding is very important since potentially confers to ablation the ability to reduce the proportion of patients requiring implantation of cardioverter defibrillators. Moreover, the authors reported that time to first AF diagnosis and heart failure diagnosis was significantly related to ablation outcome, highlighting the importance of prompt optimal treatment of both HF and AF to achieve the best clinical benefit.

http://dx.doi.org/10.5772/67024

Ganesan et al. [83], furthermore, reported meta-analyses including more than 900 patients with HF-ablated for AF showing a LVEF improvement of 13%.

Ullah et al [84] in their multicentric registry reported a significant LV ejection fraction increasing from 34.4 ± 9 to 45.8 ± 12.8% ($p < 0.001$).

One small observational prospective study specifically investigated patients with preserved LVEF [75]. This study, including 73 patients with a mean follow-up of 34 months, reported 27% efficacy after the first procedure which further raised to 73% with redo procedures and antiarrhythmic drugs. On note, LV diastolic function and systolic function measured with strain and strain rate improved only in patients maintaining stable sinus rhythm.

Moreover, data reported that effective sinus rhythm restoration after AF ablation was useful to improve LVEF in patients with tachycardiomyopathy [48, 65].

Furthermore, AF ablation in HF patients relates to a significant improvement in quality of life, functional class and exercise tolerance, which possibly relates to the improvement in LV function and hemodynamic status of the patients. In general, shorter history of HF and AF is both associated with improved outcome: AF ablation in HF patients should be considered precociously to avoid progression of atrial substrate alteration. Left atrial dimension is a marker of advanced substrate alteration; in fact, patients with severe LA dilation present lower rate of sinus rhythm maintenance.

In particular, Ullah et al. [84] reported a reduction in NYHA class from 2.3 ± 0.7 at baseline to 1.5 ± 0.8 at follow up. This was the first study to examine specifically the impact of maintaining sinus rhythm on rates of stroke and death after catheter ablation of AF patients with HF showing that restoration of sinus rhythm reduced the incidence of stroke and death (**Figure 3**).

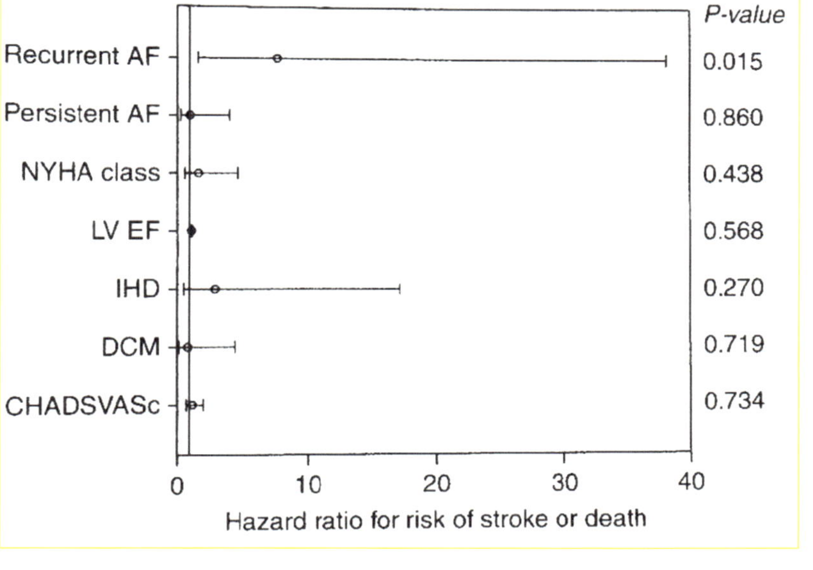

Figure 3. Factors predicting stroke and death in patients with heart failure [84].

3.3. Indications for transcatheter ablation of atrial fibrillation in patients with heart failure

Within the general population, the safety and efficacy rates of AF ablation promoted this procedure to the first choice following one antiarrhythmic drug failure and in selected patients, even the first option before drugs [1]. Its role within HF, instead, is less well defined due to small randomized trials and observational studies [48–53, 65–85]. The revised European recommendations for antiarrhythmic drug therapy leave amiodarone as the only available antiarrhythmic agent in this setting [1]. In patients who suffer from symptomatic AF recurrences on amiodarone therapy, catheter ablation remains as the sole choice for rhythm control therapy [1] (**Figure 4**). In the last guidelines, AF ablation is indicated in symptomatic patients with reduced ejection fraction in order to improve symptoms and cardiac function (class IIa, level of evidence C) [36].

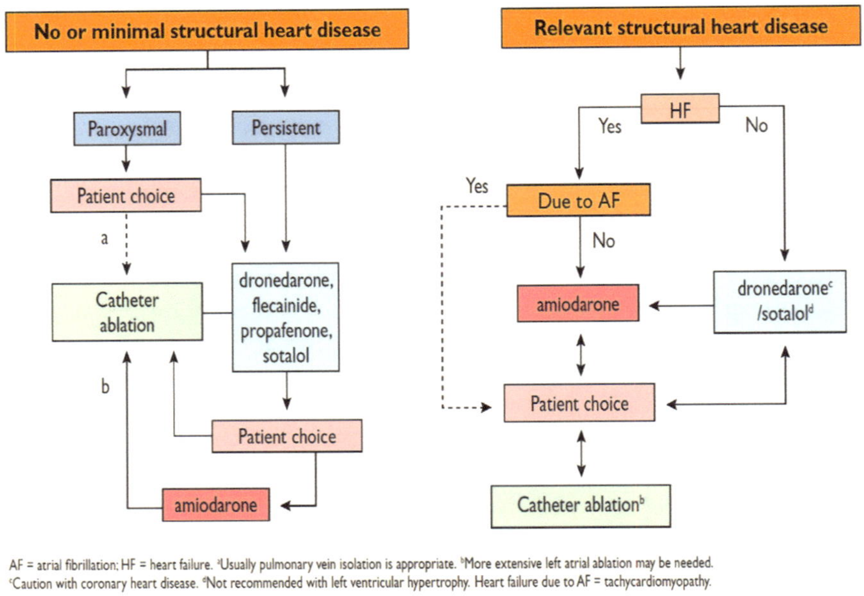

Figure 4. European Society of Cardiology guidelines for atrial fibrillation ablation [1].

3.4. Catheter ablation of atrial fibrillation in specific cardiomyopathies populations

Some observational studies reported the outcome of AF ablation among patients with hypertrophic [65, 83, 86, 88]. All studies reported low efficacy after a single ablation procedure, especially during long-term follow-up. However, the efficacy raised up to 70–80% including the over 30% redo procedures and the prevalence of extensive left atrial ablation, including linear lesions or CFAEs, which was higher when compared with the general HF population. This finding reflects a complex substrate typical of this specific cardiomyopathy, characterized by severe left atrial enlargement. Being AF detrimental on both the quality of life and prognosis of HCM patients, its effective treatment warrants careful attention and ablation may be considered precociously to achieve rhythm control.

Moreover, although AF standard treatment in valvular cardiomyopathies is more commonly surgical, performed concomitantly to heart surgery, some studies reported the outcome of AF ablation among patients with significant valvular disease. Two studies, including patients with prosthetic valves or previous percutaneous intervention for mitral rheumatic disease, reported a very low efficacy after a single procedure, raising up to 70% at a mean follow-up of 24 months including over 50% repeated procedures [87, 88]. Other two studies including patients with moderate aortic or mitral defects, instead, reported outcomes similar to the general population [87, 89].

3.5. Future perspectives

Catheter ablation of AF is gaining a significant role in HF treatment of patients with concomitant AF, as confirmed by the latest ESC guidelines. However, the following points remains of concern. First of all, pulmonary vein isolation alone and/or additional non-PV targets, as in the general population, need to be tested in prospective randomized trials on HF patients.

Further studies, moreover, should define the optimal timing to perform AF ablation in these patients to increase the success rate and reduce mortality.

In the future, technological innovations may contribute to rise AF ablation safety, for example, new irrigated catheters able to significantly reduce the fluid administration during procedure, particularly relevant among HF patients.

Finally, due to the complexity of this procedure, the suggestion is to refer to experienced, high volume centers, also skilled to manage plausible complications.

Author details

Antonio Di Monaco, Federico Quadrini, Nicola Vitulano and Massimo Grimaldi*

*Address all correspondence to: fiatric@hotmail.com

Department of Cardiology, Hospital "F. Miulli", Bari, Italy

References

[1] Camm AJ, Lip GY, De Caterina R, Savelieva I, Atar D, Hohnloser SH, Hindricks G, Kirchhof P; ESC Committee for Practice Guidelines (CPG). 2012 focused update of the ESC guidelines for the management of atrial fibrillation: an update of the 2010 ESC guidelines for the management of atrial fibrillation. Developed with the special contribution of the European Heart Rhythm Association. Eur Heart J. 2012;33:2719–2747.

[2] Schnabel RB, Yin X, Gona P, Larson MG, Beiser AS, McManus DD, Newton-Cheh C, Lubitz SA, Magnani JW, Ellinor PT, Seshadri S, Wolf PA, Vasan RS, Benjamin EJ, Levy D. 50 year trends in atrial fibrillation prevalence, incidence, risk factors and mortality in the Framingham Heart Study: a cohort study. Lancet. 2015;386:154–162.

[3] Grogan M, Smith HC, Gersh BJ, et al. Left ventricular dysfunction due to atrial fibrillation in patients initially believed to have idiopathic dilated cardiomyopathy. Am J Cardiol. 1992;69:1570–1573

[4] Kannel WB, Abbott RD, Savage DD, McNamara PM. Epidemiologic features of chronic atrial fibrillation: the Framingham study. N Engl J Med. 1982;306:1018–1022.

[5] Wolf PA, Abbott RD, Kannel WB. Atrial fibrillation as an independent risk factor for stroke: the Framingham Study. Stroke. 1991;22:983–988.

[6] Benjamin EJ, Wolf PA, D'Agostino RB,Silbershatz H, Kannel WB, Levy D.Impact of atrial fibrillation on the risk of death: the Framingham Heart Study. Circulation. 1998;98:946–952.

[7] Wyse DG, Waldo AL, DiMarco JP, Domanski MJ, Rosenberg Y, Schron EB, Kellen JC, Greene HL, Mickel MC, Dalquist JE, Corley SD; Atrial Fibrillation Follow-up Investigation of Rhythm Management (AFFIRM) Investigators. A comparison of rate control and rhythm control in patients with atrial fibrillation. N Engl J Med. 2002;347:1825–1833.

[8] Roy D, Talajic M, Nattel S, Wyse DG, Dorian P, Lee KL, Bourassa MG, Arnold JM, Buxton AE, Camm AJ, Connolly SJ, Dubuc M, Ducharme A, Guerra PG, Hohnloser SH, Lambert J, Le Heuzey JY, O'Hara G, Pedersen OD, Rouleau JL, Singh BN, Stevenson LW, Stevenson WG, Thibault B, Waldo AL; Atrial Fibrillation and Congestive Heart Failure Investigators. Rhythm control versus rate control for atrial fibrillation and heart failure. N Engl J Med. 2008;358:2667–2677.

[9] Van Gelder IC, Hagens VE, Bosker HA, Kingma JH, Kamp O, Kingma T, Said SA, Darmanata JI, Timmermans AJ, Tijssen JG, Crijns HJ; Rate Control versus Electrical Cardioversion for Persistent Atrial Fibrillation Study Group. A comparison of rate control and rhythm control in patients with recurrent persistent atrial fibrillation. N Engl J Med. 2002;347:1834–1840.

[10] Hohnloser SH, Kuck KH, Lilienthal J. Rhythm or rate control in atrial fibrillation. Pharmacological Intervention in atrial fibrillation (PIAF): a randomized trial. Lancet. 2000;356:1789–1794.

[11] Corley SD, Epstein AE, DiMarco JP, Domanski MJ, Geller N, Greene HL, Josephson RA, Kellen JC, Klein RC, Krahn AD, Mickel M, Mitchell LB, Nelson JD, Rosenberg Y, Schron E, Shemanski L, Waldo AL, Wyse DG; AFFIRM Investigators. Relationships between sinus rhythm, treatment and survival in the atrial fibrillation follow-up investigation of rhythm management (AFFIRM) study. Circulation. 2004;109:1509–1513.

[12] Hoffmann E, Sulke N, Edvardsson N, Ruiter J, Lewalter T, Capucci A, Schuchert A, Janko S, Camm J; Atrial Fibrillation Therapy Trial Investigators. New insights into the initiation of atrial fibrillation: a detailed intraindividual and interindividual analysis of the spontaneous onset of atrial fibrillation using new diagnostic pacemaker features. Circulation. 2006;113:1933–1941.

[13] Jidéus L, Kesek M, Joachimsson PO, Ericson M, Nilsson L, Blomström-Lundqvist C.The role of premature atrial contractions as the main triggers of postoperative atrial fibrillation. J Electrocardiol. 2006;39:48–54

[14] Haïssaguerre M, Jaïs P, Shah DC, Takahashi A, Hocini M, Quiniou G, Garrigue S, Le Mouroux A, Le Métayer P, Clémenty J. Spontaneous initiation of atrial fibrillation by ectopic beats originating in the pulmonary veins. N Engl J Med. 1998;339:659–666.

[15] Chen SA, Hsieh MH, Tai CT, Tsai CF, Prakash VS, Yu WC, Hsu TL, Ding YA, Chang MS. Initiation of atrial fibrillation by ectopic beats originating from the pulmonary veins: electrophysiological characteristics, pharmacological responses and effects of radiofrequency ablation. Circulation. 1999;100:1879–1886.

[16] Valles E, Fan R, Roux JF, Liu CF, Harding JD, Dhruvakumar S, Hutchinson MD, Riley M, Bala R, Garcia FC, Lin D, Dixit S, Callans DJ, Gerstenfeld EP, Marchlinski FE. Localization of atrial fibrillation triggers in patients undergoing pulmonary vein isolation: importance of the carina region. J Am Coll Cardiol. 2008;52:1413–1420.

[17] Hocini M, Haïssaguerre M, Shah D, Jaïs P, Peng JT, Yamane T, Deisenhofer I, Garrigue S, Fuimaono K, Pike R, Clémenty J. Multiple sources initiating atrial fibrillation from a single pulmonary vein identified by a circumferential catheter. Pacing Clin Electrophysiol. 2000;23:1828–1831.

[18] Haïssaguerre M, Jaïs P, Shah DC, Garrigue S, Takahashi A, Lavergne T, Hocini M, Peng JT, Roudaut R, Clémenty J. Electrophysiological end point for catheter ablation of atrial fibrillation initiated from multiple pulmonary venous foci. Circulation. 2000;101:1409–1417

[19] Ouyang F, Bänsch D, Ernst S, Schaumann A, Hachiya H, Chen M, Chun J, Falk P, Khanedani A, Antz M, Kuck KH. Complete isolation of left atrium surrounding the pulmonary veins: new insights from the double-Lasso technique in paroxysmal atrial fibrillation. Circulation. 2004;110:2090–2096.

[20] Weerasooriya R, Jaïs P, Scavée C, Macle L, Shah DC, Arentz T, Salerno JA, Raybaud F, Choi KJ, Hocini M, Clémenty J, Haïssaguerre M. Dissociated pulmonary vein arrhythmia: incidence and characteristics. J Cardiovasc Electrophysiol. 2003;14:1173–1179.

[21] Jaïs P, Haïssaguerre M, Shah DC, Chouairi S, Gencel L, Hocini M, Clémenty J. A focal source of atrial fibrillation treated by discrete radiofrequency ablation. Circulation. 1997;95:572–576.

[22] Kumagai K, Yasuda T, Tojo H, Noguchi H, Matsumoto N, Nakashima H, Gondo N, Saku K. Role of rapid focal activation in the maintenance of atrial fibrillation originating from the pulmonary veins. Pacing Clin Electrophysiol. 2000;23:1823–1827.

[23] O'Donnell D, Furniss SS, Bourke JP. Paroxysmal cycle length shortening in the pulmonary veins during atrial fibrillation correlates with arrhythmogenic triggering foci in sinus rhythm. J Cardiovasc Electrophysiol. 2002;13:124–128.

[24] Oral H, Ozaydin M, Tada H, Chugh A, Scharf C, Hassan S, Lai S, Greenstein R, Pelosi F Jr, Knight BP, Strickberger SA, Morady F. Mechanistic significance of intermittent pulmonary vein tachycardia in patients with atrial fibrillation. J Cardiovasc Electrophysiol. 2002;13:645–650.

[25] Nault I, Wright M, Hocini M, Haïssaguerre M, Jaïs P. Extreme firing in a pulmonary vein during atrial fibrillation. J Cardiovasc Electrophysiol 2009;20:696.

[26] Haïssaguerre M, Sanders P, Hocini M, Hsu LF, Shah DC, Scavée C, Takahashi Y, Rotter M, Pasquié JL, Garrigue S, Clémenty J, Jaïs P. Changes in atrial fibrillation cycle length and inducibility during catheter ablation and their relation to outcome. Circulation. 2004;109:3007–3013.

[27] Haïssaguerre M, Sanders P, Hocini M, Jaïs P, Clémenty J. Pulmonary veins in the substrate for atrial fibrillation: the "venous wave" hypothesis. J Am Coll Cardiol. 2004;43:2290–2292.

[28] Sanders P, Berenfeld O, Hocini M, Jaïs P, Vaidyanathan R, Hsu LF, Garrigue S, Takahashi Y, Rotter M, Sacher F, Scavée C, Ploutz-Snyder R, Jalife J, Haïssaguerre M. Spectral analysis identifies sites of high-frequency activity maintaining atrial fibrillation in humans. Circulation. 2005;112:789–797.

[29] Marrouche NF, Wilber D, Hindricks G, Jais P, Akoum N, Marchlinski F, Kholmovski E, Burgon N, Hu N, Mont L, Deneke T, Duytschaever M, Neumann T, Mansour M, Mahnkopf C, Herweg B, Daoud E, Wissner E, Bansmann P, Brachmann J. Association of atrial tissue fibrosis identified by delayed enhancement MRI and atrial fibrillation catheter ablation: the DECAAF study. JAMA. 2014;311:498–506.

[30] Eckstein J, Zeemering S, Linz D, Maesen B, Verheule S, van Hunnik A, Crijns H, Allessie MA, Schotten U. Transmural conduction is the predominant mechanism of breakthrough during atrial fibrillation: evidence from simultaneous endo-epicardial high-density activation mapping. Circ Arrhythm Electrophysiol. 2013;6:334–341.

[31] Rewiuk K, Wizner B, Fedyk-Lukasik M, Zdrojewski T, Opolski G, Dubiel JS, Grodzicki T. The growing rate of atrial fibrillation among heart failure patients in polish primary health care - data from 2005 and 2013. J Hypertens. 2016;34:e23.

[32] Li SJ, Sartipy U, Lund LH, Dahlström U, Adiels M, Petzold M, Fu M. Prognostic significance of resting heart rate and use of β-blockers in atrial fibrillation and sinus rhythm in patients with heart failure and reduced ejection fraction: findings from the Swedish Heart Failure Registry. Circ Heart Fail. 2015;8:871–879.

[33] Mareev Y, Cleland JGF. Should β-blockers be used in patients with heart failure and atrial fibrillation? Clin Ther. 2015;37:2215–2224.

[34] Van Gelder IC, Wyse DG, Chandler ML, Cooper HA, Olshansky B, Hagens VE, Crijns HJ; RACE and AFFIRM Investigators. Does intensity of rate-control influence outcome in atrial fibrillation? An analysis of pooled data from the RACE and AFFIRM studies. Europace. 2006;8:935–942.

http://dx.doi.org/10.5772/67024

[35] Van Gelder IC, Groenveld HF, Crijns HJGM, Tuininga YS, Tijssen JGP, Alings AM, Hillege HL, Bergsma-Kadijk JA, Cornel JH, Kamp O, Tukkie R, Bosker HA, Van Veldhuisen DJ, Van den Berg MP, RACE II Investigators. Lenient versus strict rate control in patients with atrial fibrillation. N Engl J Med. 2010;362:1363 – 1373.

[36] Kirchhof P, Benussi S, Kotecha D, Ahlsson A, Atar D, Casadei B, Castella M, Diener HC, Heidbuchel H, Hendriks J, Hindricks G, Manolis AS, Oldgren J, Popescu BA, Schotten U, Van Putte B, Vardas P, Agewall S, Camm J, Baron Esquivias G, Budts W, Carerj S, Casselman F, Coca A, De Caterina R, Deftereos S, Dobrev D, Ferro JM, Filippatos G, Fitzsimons D, Gorenek B, Guenoun M, Hohnloser SH, Kolh P, Lip GY, Manolis A, McMurray J, Ponikowski P, Rosenhek R, Ruschitzka F, Savelieva I, Sharma S, Suwalski P, Tamargo JL, Taylor CJ, Van Gelder IC, Voors AA, Windecker S, Zamorano JL, Zeppenfeld K. 2016 ESC Guidelines for the management of atrial fibrillation developed in collaboration with EACTS. Eur Heart J 2016;37:2893–2962.

[37] Kotecha D, Holmes J, Krum H, Altman DG, Manzano L, Cleland JGF, Lip GYH, Coats AJS, Andersson B, Kirchhof P, von Lueder TG, Wedel H, Rosano G, Shibata MC, Rigby A, Flather MD. Efficacy of β blockers in patients with heart failure plus atrial fibrillation: an individual-patient data meta-analysis. Lancet. 2014; 384:2235– 2243.

[38] Allen LA, Fonarow GC, Simon DN, Thomas LE, Marzec LN, Pokorney SD, Gersh BJ, Go AS, Hylek EM, Kowey PR, Mahaffey KW, Chang P, Peterson ED, Piccini JP. Digoxin use and subsequent outcomes among patients in a contemporary atrial fibrillation cohort. J Am Coll Cardiol 2015;65:2691–2698.

[39] Gheorghiade M, Fonarow GC, van Veldhuisen DJ, Cleland JGF, Butler J, Epstein AE, Patel K, Aban IB, Aronow WS, Anker SD, Ahmed A. Lack of evidence of increased mortality among patients with atrial fibrillation taking digoxin: findings from post hoc propensity-matched analysis of the AFFIRM trial. Eur Heart J. 2013;34:1489–1497.

[40] Turakhia MP, Santangeli P, Winkelmayer WC, Xu X, Ullal AJ, Than CT, Schmitt S, Holmes TH, Frayne SM, Phibbs CS, Yang F, Hoang DD, Ho PM, Heidenreich PA. Increased mortality associated with digoxin in contemporary patients with atrial fibrillation. J Am Coll Cardiol. 2014;64:660–668.

[41] Carlsson J, Miketic S, Windeler J, et al. STAF Investigators. Randomized trial of rate control versus rhythm control in persistent atrial fibrillation: the strategies of treatment in atrial fibrillation (STAF) Study. J Am Coll Cardiol. 2003;41:1690–1696.

[42] Opolski G, Torbicki A, Kosior D, et al. Rhythm control versus rate control in patients with persistent atrial fibrillation. Results of the HOT CAFE Polish study. Pol Heart J. 2003;59:15–16.

[43] The AFFIRM Investigators. Relationships between sinus rhythm, treatment and survival in the atrial fibrillation follow-up investigation of rhythm management (AFFIRM) study. Circulation. 2004;109:1509–1513.

[44] Olshansky B, Rosenfeld LE, Warner AK; AFFIRM Investigators. The atrial fibrillation follow-up investigation of rhythm management (AFFIRM) study: approaches to control rate in atrial fibrillation. J Am Coll Cardiol. 2004;43:1201–1208.

[45] Brignole M, Menozzi C, Gianfranchi L, et al. Assessment of atrioventricular junction ablation and VVIR pacemaker versus pharmacological treatment in patients with heart failure and chronic atrial fibrillation: a randomized, controlled study. Circulation. 1998;98:953–960.

[46] Roy D, Talajic M, Dorian P, et al., Canadian Trial of Atrial Fibrillation Investigators. Amiodarone to prevent recurrence of atrial fibrillation. N Engl J Med. 2000;342:913–920.

[47] Deedwania PC, Singh BN, Ellenbogen K, et al. for the Department of Veterans Affairs CHF-STAT Investigators. Spontaneous conversion and maintenance of sinus rhythm by amiodarone in patients with heart failure and atrial fibrillation: observations from the veterans affairs congestive heart failure survival trial of antiarrhythmic therapy (CHF-STAT). Circulation. 1998;98:2574–2579.

[48] Choi AD, Hematpour K, Kukin M, Mittal S, Steinberg JS. Ablation vs medical therapy in the setting of symptomatic atrial fibrillation and left ventricular dysfunction. Congest Heart Fail. 2010;16:10–14.

[49] Gentlesk PJ, Sauer WH, Gerstenfeld EP, Lin D, Dixit S, Zado E, Callans D, Marchlinski FE. Reversal of left ventricular dysfunction following ablation of atrial fibrillation. J Cardiovasc Electrophysiol. 2007;18:9–14.

[50] Hsu LF, Jaïs P, Sanders P, Garrigue S, Hocini M, Sacher F, Takahashi Y, Rotter M, Pasquié JL, Scavée C, Bordachar P, Clémenty J, Haïssaguerre M. Catheter ablation for atrial fibrillation in congestive heart failure. N Engl J Med. 2004;351:2373–2383.

[51] Tondo C, Mantica M, Russo G, Avella A, De Luca L, Pappalardo A, Fagundes RL, Picchio E, Laurenzi F, Piazza V, Bisceglia I. Pulmonary vein vestibule ablation for the control of atrial fibrillation in patients with impaired left ventricular function. Pacing Clin Electrophysiol. 2006;29:962–970.

[52] MacDonald MR, Connelly DT, Hawkins NM, Steedman T, Payne J, Shaw M, Denvir M, Bhagra S, Small S, Martin W, McMurray JJ, Petrie MC. Radio-frequency ablation for persistent atrial fibrillation in patients with advanced heart failure and severe left ventricular systolic dysfunction: a randomized controlled trial. Heart. 2011;97:740–747.

[53] Wilton SB, Fundytus A, Ghali WA, Veenhuyzen GD, Quinn FR, Mitchell LB, Hill MD, Faris P, Exner DV. Meta-analysis of the effectiveness and safety of catheter ablation of atrial fibrillation in patients with versus without left ventricular systolic dysfunction. Am J Cardiol. 2010;106:1284–1291.

[54] Lin WS, Tai CT, Hsieh MH, Tsai CF, Lin YK, Tsao HM, Huang JL, Yu WC, Yang SP, Ding YA, Chang MS, Chen SA. Catheter ablation of paroxysmal atrial fibrillation initiated by non-pulmonary vein ectopy. Circulation. 2003;107:3176–3183.

[55] Yamaguchi T, Tsuchiya T, Miyamoto K, Nagamoto Y, Takahashi N. Characterization of non-pulmonary vein foci with an EnSite array in patients with paroxysmal atrial fibrillation. Europace. 2010;12:1698–1706.

[56] Chen SA, Tai CT. Catheter ablation of atrial fibrillation originating from the non-pulmonary vein foci. J Cardiovasc Electrophysiol. 2005;16:229–232.

[57] Patel D, Mohanty P, Di Biase L, et al. Outcomes and complications of catheter ablation for atrial fibrillation in females. Heart Rhythm. 2010;7:167–172.

[58] Santangeli P, Di Biase L, Mohanty P, et al. Catheter ablation of atrial fibrillation in octogenarians: safety and outcomes. J Cardiovasc Electrophysiol. 2012;23:687–693.

[59] Takigawa M, Kuwahara T, Takahashi A, et al. Differences in catheter ablation of paroxysmal atrial fibrillation between males and females. Int J Cardiol. 2013;168:1984–1991.

[60] Elayi CS, DI Biase L, Bai R, et al. Administration of isoproterenol and adenosine to guide supplemental ablation after pulmonary vein antrum isolation. J Cardiovasc Electrophysiol. 2013;24:1199–1206.

[61] Zhao Y, Di Biase L, Trivedi C, et al. Importance of non-pulmonary vein triggers ablation to achieve long-term freedom from paroxysmal atrial fibrillation in patients with low ejection fraction. Heart Rhythm. 2016;13:141–149.

[62] Allessie M, Ausma J, Schotten U. Electrical, contractile and structural remodeling during atrial fibrillation. Cardiovasc Res. 2002;54:230–246.

[63] Knecht S, Hocini M, Wright M, Lellouche N, O'Neill MD, Matsuo S et al. Left atrial linear lesions are required for successful treatment of persistent atrial fibrillation. Eur Heart J. 2008;29:2359–2366.

[64] Tamborero D, Mont L, Berruezo A, Matiello M, Benito B, Sitges M et al. Left atrial posterior wall isolation does not improve the outcome of circumferential pulmonary vein ablation for atrial fibrillation: a prospective randomized study. Circ Arrhythm Electrophysiol. 2009;2:35–40.

[65] Anselmino M, Matta M, D'Ascenzo F, Bunch TJ, Schilling RJ, Hunter RJ, Pappone C, Neumann T, Noelker G, Fiala M, Bertaglia E, Frontera A, Duncan E, Nalliah C, Jais P, Weerasooriya R, Kalman JM, Gaita F. Catheter ablation of atrial fibrillation in patients with left ventricular systolic dysfunction: a systematic review and meta-analysis. Circ Arrhythm Electrophysiol. 2014;7:1011–1118.

[66] Chen MS, Marrouche NF, Khaykin Y, Gillinov AM, Wazni O, Martin DO, Rossillo A, Verma A, Cummings J, Erciyes D, Saad E, Bhargava M, Bash D, Schweikert R, Burkhardt D, Williams-Andrews M, Perez-Lugones A, Abdul-Karim A, Saliba W, Natale A. Pulmonary vein isolation for the treatment of atrial fibrillation in patients with impaired systolic function. J Am Coll Cardiol. 2004;43:1004–1009.

[67] Efremidis M, Sideris A, Xydonas S, Letsas KP, Alexanian IP, Manolatos D, Mihas CC, Filippatos GS, Kardaras F. Ablation of atrial fibrillation in patients with heart failure: reversal of atrial and ventricular remodelling. Hellenic J Cardiol. 2008;49:19–25

[68] Nademanee K, Schwab MC, Kosar EM, Karwecki M, Moran MD, Visessook N, Michael AD, Ngarmukos T. Clinical outcomes of catheter substrate ablation for high-risk patients with atrial fibrillation. J Am Coll Cardiol. 2008;51:843–849.

[69] Lutomsky BA, Rostock T, Koops A, Steven D, Müllerleile K, Servatius H, Drewitz I, Ueberschär D, Plagemann T, Ventura R, Meinertz T, Willems S. Catheter ablation of paroxysmal atrial fibrillation improves cardiac function: a prospective study on the impact of atrial fibrillation ablation on left ventricular function assessed by magnetic resonance imaging. Europace. 2008;10:593–599.

[70] De Potter T, Berruezo A, Mont L, Matiello M, Tamborero D, Santibañez C, Benito B, Zamorano N, Brugada J. Left ventricular systolic dysfunction by itself does not influence outcome of atrial fibrillation ablation. Europace. 2010;12:24–29

[71] Cha YM, Wokhlu A, Asirvatham SJ, Shen WK, Friedman PA, Munger TM, Oh JK, Monahan KH, Haroldson JM, Hodge DO, Herges RM, Hammill SC, Packer DL Success of ablation for atrial fibrillation in isolated left ventricular diastolic dysfunction: a comparison to systolic dysfunction and normal ventricular function. Circ Arrhythm Electrophysiol. 2011;4:724–732.

[72] Anselmino M, Grossi S, Scaglione M, Castagno D, Bianchi F, Senatore G, Matta M, Casolati D, Ferraris F, Cristoforetti Y, Negro A, Gaita F. Long-term results of transcatheter atrial fibrillation ablation in patients with impaired left ventricular systolic function. J Cardiovasc Electrophysiol. 2013;24:24–32.

[73] Calvo N, Bisbal F, Guiu E, Ramos P, Nadal M, Tolosana JM, Arbelo E, Berruezo A, Sitges M, Brugada J, Mont L. Impact of atrial fibrillation-induced tachycardiomyopathy in patients undergoing pulmonary vein isolation. Int J Cardiol. 2013;168:4093–4097.

[74] Nedios S, Sommer P, Dagres N, Kosiuk J, Arya A, Richter S, Gaspar T, Kanagkinis N, Dinov B, Piorkowski C, Bollmann A, Hindricks G, Rolf S. Long-term follow-up after atrial fibrillation ablation in patients with impaired left ventricular systolic function: the importance of rhythm and rate control. Heart Rhythm. 2014;11:344–351.

[75] Kosiuk J, Nedios S, Darma A, Rolf S, Richter S, Arya A, Piorkowski C, Gaspar T, Sommer P, Husser D, Hindricks G, Bollmann A. Impact of single atrial fibrillation catheter ablation on implantable cardioverter defibrillator therapies in patients with ischaemic and non-ischaemic cardiomyopathies. Europace. 2014;16:1322–1326.

[76] Lobo TJ, Pachon CT, Pachon JC, Pachon EI, Pachon MZ, Pachon JC, Santillana TG, Zerpa JC, Albornoz RN, Jatene AD. Atrial fibrillation ablation in systolic dysfunction: clinical and echocardiographic outcomes. Arq Bras Cardiol. 2015;104:45–52.

[77] Bunch TJ, May HT, Bair TL, Jacobs V, Crandall BG, Cutler M, Weiss JP, Mallender C, Osborn JS, Anderson JL, Day JD. Five-year outcomes of catheter ablation in patients with atrial fibrillation and left ventricular systolic dysfunction. J Cardiovasc Electrophysiol. 2015;26:363–370.

[78] Machino-Ohtsuka T, Seo Y, Ishizu T, Sugano A, Atsumi A, Yamamoto M, Kawamura R, Machino T, Kuroki K, Yamasaki H, Igarashi M, Sekiguchi Y, Aonuma K. Efficacy, safety and outcomes of catheter ablation of atrial fibrillation in patients with heart failure with preserved ejection fraction. J Am Coll Cardiol. 2013;62:1857–1865.

[79] Khan MN, Jaïs P, Cummings J, Di Biase L, Sanders P, Martin DO, Kautzner J, Hao S, Themistoclakis S, Fanelli R, Potenza D, Massaro R, Wazni O, Schweikert R, Saliba W, Wang P, Al-Ahmad A, Beheiry S, Santarelli P, Starling RC, Dello Russo A, Pelargonio G, Brachmann J, Schibgilla V, Bonso A, Casella M, Raviele A, Haïssaguerre M, Natale A; PABA-CHF Investigators. Pulmonary-vein isolation for atrial fibrillation in patients with heart failure. N Engl J Med. 2008;359:1778–1785.

[80] Jones DG, Haldar SK, Hussain W, Sharma R, Francis DP, Rahman-Haley SL, McDonagh TA, Underwood SR, Markides V, Wong T. A randomized trial to assess catheter ablation versus rate control in the management of persistent atrial fibrillation in heart failure. J Am Coll Cardiol. 2013;61:1894–1903.

[81] Hunter RJ, Berriman TJ, Diab I, Kamdar R, Richmond L, Baker V, Goromonzi F, Sawhney V, Duncan E, Page SP, Ullah W, Unsworth B, Mayet J, Dhinoja M, Earley MJ, Sporton S, Schilling RJ. A randomized controlled trial of catheter ablation versus medical treatment of atrial fibrillation in heart failure (the CAMTAF trial). Circ Arrhythm Electrophysiol. 2014;7:31–38.

[82] Dagres N, Varounis C, Gaspar T, Piorkowski C, Eitel C, Iliodromitis EK, Lekakis JP, Flevari P, Simeonidou E, Rallidis LS, Tsougos E, Hindricks G, Sommer P, Anastasiou-Nana M. Catheter ablation for atrial fibrillation in patients with left ventricular systolic dysfunction. A systematic review and meta-analysis. J Card Fail. 2011;17:964–970.

[83] Ganesan AN, Nandal S, Lüker J, Pathak RK, Mahajan R, Twomey D, Lau DH, Sanders P. Catheter ablation of atrial fibrillation in patients with concomitant left ventricular impairment: a systematic review of efficacy and effect on ejection fraction. Heart Lung Circ. 2015;24:270–280.

[84] Ullah W, Ling LH, Prabhu S, Lee G, Kistler P, Finlay MC, Earley MJ, Sporton S, Bashir Y, Betts TR, Rajappan K, Thomas G, Duncan E, Staniforth A, Mann I, Chow A, Lambiase P, Schilling RJ, Hunter RJ. Catheter ablation of atrial fibrillation in patients with heart failure: impact of maintaining sinus rhythm on heart failure status and long-term rates of stroke and death. Europace. 2016;18:679–686.

[85] Zhu M, Zhou X, Cai H, Wang Z, Xu H, Chen S, Chen J, Xu X, Xu H, Mao W. Catheter ablation versus medical rate control for persistent atrial fibrillation in patients with heart failure: a PRISMA-compliant systematic review and meta-analysis of randomized controlled trials. Medicine (Baltimore). 2016;95:e4377.

[86] Santangeli P, Di Biase L, Themistoclakis S, Raviele A, Schweikert RA, Lakkireddy D, Mohanty P, Bai R, Mohanty S, Pump A, Beheiry S, Hongo R, Sanchez JE, Gallinghouse GJ, Horton R, Dello Russo A, Casella M, Fassini G, Elayi CS, Burkhardt JD, Tondo C, Natale A. Catheter ablation of atrial fibrillation in hypertrophic cardiomyopathy: long-term outcomes and mechanisms of arrhythmia recurrence. Circ Arrhythm Electrophysiol. 2013;6:1089–1094.

[87] Khaykin Y, Marrouche NF, Saliba W, Schweikert R, Bash D, Chen MS, Williams-Andrews M, Saad E, Burkhardt DJ, Bhargava M, Joseph G, Rossillo A, Erciyes D, Martin D, Natale A. Pulmonary vein antrum isolation for treatment of atrial fibrillation in patients with valvular heart disease or prior open heart surgery. Heart Rhythm. 2004;1:33–39.

[88] Wang X, Liu X, Shi H, Gu J, Sun Y, Zhou L, Hu W. Heart rhythm disorders and pacemakers: pulmonary vein isolation combined with substrate modification for persistent atrial fibrillation treatment in patients with valvular heart diseases. Heart. 2009;95:1773–1783.

[89] Okamatsu H, Ohara T, Kanzaki H, Nakajima I, Miyamoto K, Okamura H, Noda T, Aiba T, Kusano K, Kamakura S, Shimizu W, Satomi K. Impact of left ventricular diastolic dysfunction on outcome of catheter ablation for atrial fibrillation in patients with hypertrophic cardiomyopathy. Circ J. 2015;79:419–424.

Chapter 7

Role of the Electrophysiologist in the Treatment of Tachycardia-Induced Cardiomyopathy

Cismaru Gabriel, Lucian Muresan, Puiu Mihai,
Radu Rosu, Gabriel Gusetu, Dana Pop and
Dumitru Zdrenghea

Additional information is available at the end of the chapter

http://dx.doi.org/10.5772/66515

Abstract

Tachycardia-induced cardiomyopathy is a systolic cardiac dysfunction given by prolonged elevated heart rates in patients with incessant or frequent tachyarrhythmias. Arrhythmias associated with tachycardiomyopathy can be either supraventricular (atrial tachycardia, atrial flutter, atrial fibrillation, AVNRT, permanent junctional reciprocating tachycardia, high rates of atrial pacing) or ventricular (frequent premature ventricular complexes, right ventricular outflow tract tachycardia, LVOT, left ventricular fascicular tachycardia, bundle-branch reentry or high rate of ventricular pacing). Electrophysiological study confirms the clinical diagnosis of tachycardia-induced cardiomyopathy, reveals the arrhythmia mechanism and facilitates catheter ablation that results in complete recovery of ventricular function. This chapter has two parts: 1. **Theoretical insight** into the pathogenesis of tachycardia-induced cardiomyopathy, clinical manifestations and therapy. 2. **Practical issues**: we describe our EP lab's experience on electrophysiological study and ablation in patients with tachycardia-induced cardiomyopathy. We will present five cases of ablation: PVCs >30,000/24 h, antidromic tachycardia, 2:1 atrial flutter, persistent atrial fibrillation and RVOT PVCs with nonsustained VT.

Keywords: catheter ablation, tachycardia-induced cardiomyopathy, atrial fibrillation, ejection fraction, left ventricular dysfunction

1. Introduction

Cardiomyopathy is defined by a disease of the heart muscle that progressively worsens and ultimately leads to heart failure and death. Fortunately, there are some reversible cardiomyopathies that can show return to normal cardiac function with or without treatment: peripartum cardiomyopathy, myocarditis with dilated cardiomyopathy, hyperthyroidism-induced cardiomyopathy, takotsubo cardiomyopathy and tachycardia-induced cardiomyopathy. The last one is a disease caused by a persistent tachycardia with return to normal cardiac function after correction of the arrhythmia.

Arrhythmias that are associated with this type of reversible cardiomyopathy include atrial fibrillation, atrial flutter, atrial tachycardia, atrioventricular node reentrant tachycardia, accessory pathway tachycardia, frequent ventricular ectopic beats and ventricular tachycardia.

2. Experimental studies on animals

Animal models helped us to better evaluate cellular and hemodynamic mechanisms underlying tachycardia-induced cardiomyopathy. Whipple et al. described it in an interesting experiment on dogs and pigs using cardiac pacing. Chronic rapid ventricular pacing leads to left biventricular dilatation and decreases in systolic function. When pacing at slower rate or for shorter duration, the degree of dilatation is not so important, as well as the decrease in ejection fraction. Mitral regurgitation appears as a consequence of left ventricular dilatation [1].

3. Clinical studies on humans

Multiple tachyarrhythmias have been associated with tachycardia-induced cardiomyopathy including supraventricular and ventricular. Additionally, premature ventricular beats have also been associated with the development of tachycardia-induced cardiomyopathy.

Gentlesk et al. noted that ablation of arrhythmia with restoration of sinus rhythm can improve LV function despite good rate control before the ablation procedure in patients with atrial fibrillation [2]. The most recent series of patients with incessant atrial tachycardia reported normalization of left ventricular function in 97% of the patients after successful ablation [3]. Incessant reentrant supraventricular tachycardias are less common, but tachycardia-induced cardiomyopathy has also been reported in the settings of atrioventricular node reentrant tachycardia, atrioventricular tachycardia using an accessory pathway and permanent junctional form of reentrant tachycardia [4]. When VT leads to tachycardia-induced cardiomyopathy, it is generally idiopathic, originating from RVOT, LVOT or coronary cusps. Premature ventricular contractions have also been associated with the disease.

Medi et al. identified variables associated with tachycardia-induced cardiomyopathy: incessant tachycardia, male gender, mean ventricular rate above 117 bpm and tachycardia originating from the pulmonary veins or left/right appendage [3].

In recent studies, electrical remodeling was demonstrated to precede structural remodeling with subsequent clinical adverse outcomes. In DAVID trial [5], ventricular pacing was associated with increased rate of heart failure hospitalization and cardiac mortality. The trial was designed to test the hypothesis that physiologic heart rates obtained with beta-blockers during ventricular pacing improve survival in patients with heart failure. Contrary to logical thinking,

http://dx.doi.org/10.5772/66515

ventricular pacing had higher incidence of heart failure and cardiac mortality as mentioned above. Recent therapeutic advances using biventricular pacing aim to synchronize electrical activation of the left and right ventricle and reverse structural remodeling. This approach may be of use for tachycardia-induced cardiomyopathy in patients with ventricular pacing or ventricular premature contractions (left ventricular pacing triggered by right ventricular PVCs) but not for tachyarrhythmias [6].

4. Structural changes

Sustained ventricular or atrial pacing leads to dilatation of all cardiac chambers with systolic and diastolic dysfunction. Cardiac dilatation is accompanied by ventricular wall thinning and elevated ventricular filling pressures with reduced cardiac output. Mitral valve regurgitation appears as a consequence of left ventricular dilatation and stretching of the mitral chordae and annulus [7].

5. Neurohormonal changes

Low cardiac output leads to neurohormonal activation with elevated plasma catecholamines, atrial natriuretic peptide, rennin and aldosterone [8].

6. Cellular changes

At the cellular level, it has been found that chronic rapid heart rate causes increase in myocite length and disruption of the sarcolemmal membrane interface, impairing myocardial function [9]. Abnormalities of the sarcoplasmic reticulum calcium transport may appear at 24 h after initiation of rapid atrial pacing and persist 4 weeks after cessation of pacing. The lower availability of calcium to myocites may reduce contractility [10]. Besides myocardial energy depletion, myocardial ischemia has been proposed as a possible mechanism for myocardial systolic dysfunction.

7. Tachycardia-induced cardiomyopathy and post-tachycardia T-wave memory

Both post-tachycardia T-wave memory and tachycardia-induced cardiomyopathy are two phenomenon characterized by electrical remodeling of the ventricles that occur after sustained episodes of tachyarrhythmias.

In cardiac memory, the hallmark is diffuse T-wave inversion. It also appears after persistent abnormal ventricular conduction such as ventricular pacing, intermittent bundle-branch block or ventricular preexcitation. This phenomenon was described in early 1940s in patients with ventricular tachyarrhythmias, but the term of cardiac memory was first introduced by Rosenbaum in 1982 [11]. Abnormal ventricular activation causes change in the action potential duration in the early versus late activated regions of the myocardium that results in increased transmural repolarization gradient. The duration of inverse T-wave polarity is related to the duration of abnormal ventricular conduction and may have short-term or long-term persistence.

The time course of tachycardia-induced cardiomyopathy can be variable: days to months and even years. It is not known why some patients respond to persistent tachycardia with dilation of the heart chambers and others by negativation of T-waves.

T-wave inversion lasting minutes to hours are described as short-term memory and are observed after short episodes of tachyarrhythmias. Long-term memory lasts hours to days and occurs after temporary cessation of a permanent pacing or after a successful ablation of an accessory pathway. Previous reported cases of transient T-wave inversion following tachycardia failed to show an association between duration of the tachycardia and magnitude and duration of the T-wave changes. Freundlich reported an episode of ventricular tachycardia lasting 10 min and followed by T-wave inversion for 3 weeks [12]. Dubbs and Parmet described a case of VT lasting 21 days and followed by T-wave inversion for only 4 days [13]. Campbell reported a case of atrial tachycardia with a duration of 3 days followed by T-wave inversion for other 3 days [14].

8. Time course and recovery of the LV function

The time course of reversal can be variable and may vary from 1 day to several months and even years [15]. The factors that determine the improvement rate remain undefined. It is a combination of genetic and structural heart disease factors that determine the development of the tachycardia-induced cardiomyopathy.

Han et al. [15] reported a patient with dramatic improvement of the LV systolic function <24 h after ablation with improvement of symptoms of congestion the first day after ablation.

Chin et al. [16] reported a series of patients who had improvement of the ejection fraction after 6 months of rate control: two patients with atrial fibrillation treated for heart rate control, two patients with atrial tachycardia treated for heart rate control and two patients with severe systolic dysfunction EF < 20% and recovery of systolic function after adequate treatment. The "slower" the rate control of the tachycardia, the slower the rate of improvement of the systolic function of the left ventricle. In contrast, patients with very low ejection fraction <20% have a slower rate of improvement. Chin et al. evaluated systolic function using either echocardiography or radionuclide angiography [16]. Danadamudi et al. reported patients with ejection fraction normalization after 14 months, but elevated left ventricular end-systolic and end-diastolic volume indexes were still present at follow-up.

9. Risk of recurrence

In patients with prior history of tachycardia-induced cardiomyopathy, recurrence of the arrhythmia leads to a more severe form compared to the initial presentation [17].

http://dx.doi.org/10.5772/66515

10. Clinical features and diagnostic considerations

Arrhythmias associated with tachycardiomyopathy can be supraventricular (atrial tachycardia, atrial flutter, atrial fibrillation, AVNRT, permanent junctional reciprocating tachycardia, high rates of atrial pacing) or ventricular (frequent premature ventricular complexes, right ventricular outflow tract tachycardia, LVOT, left ventricular fascicular tachycardia, bundle-branch reentry or high rate of ventricular pacing).

The exact incidence of the disease is difficult to assess, as the most reports in medical literature are small retrospective series or case studies.

Tachycardia-induced cardiomyopathy occurs independent of the age: it is present in children [18], adolescents [19], adults [20] and aged persons [21]. In children and adolescents, it should be differentiated form dilated cardiomyopathy due to myocarditis. In this case, cardiac MRI and cardiac biopsy are required to confirm the diagnosis. In adults, other forms of reversible cardiomyopathies should be excluded as follows: peripartum cardiomyopathy, myocarditis with dilated cardiomyopathy, hyperthyroidism-induced cardiomyopathy and takotsubo cardiomyopathy. The time course of the cardiomyopathy and lack of arrhythmia can exclude tachycardia-induced cardiomyopathy. Paraclinical examinations contribute to the differential diagnosis. In aged persons, idiopathic dilated cardiomyopathy is the main differential diagnosis and the presence of a sustained arrhythmia other than sinus rhythm leads to the correct diagnosis.

There is no specific test for the diagnosis of tachycardia-induced cardiomyopathy. A clinical index of suspicion derives from history of symptoms and signs of heart failure and time course of arrhythmia. Therefore, a high index of suspicion should be considered in any patient with sustained tachyarrhythmia and dilated cardiomyopathy and depressed ejection fraction. Any prolonged rate above 120/min may be important for the diagnosis. Patients may develop tachycardia-induced cardiomyopathy even if well-controlled heart rates during rest and high ventricular rate during minimal activity [22]. Holter monitoring on 24 h may be useful in assessing heart rates during minimal exertion or daily physical activity in patients with persistent atrial fibrillation [23].

11. Imaging studies in tachycardia-induced cardiomyopathy

Echocardiography is the cornerstone of the noninvasive imaging of tachycardia-induced cardiomyopathy. Increase in ejection fraction after arrhythmia treatment with decrease in ventricular diameters is diagnostic for the disease.

Radionuclide ventriculography is another noninvasive diagnostic technique showing left and right ventricular dilatation and systolic dysfunction.

Cardiac MRI identifies areas of myocardial fibrosis. Hasdemir et al. demonstrated lack of fibrosis in 18 out of 19 patients with tachycardia-induced cardiomyopathy. They concluded that PVC-induced cardiomyopathy is less likely to evaluate with fibrosis [24]. This study is consistent with the findings of Redfield et al. who demonstrated in a canine model that inflammation, fibrosis and mitochondrial apoptosis are absent in PVC-induced cardiomyopathy [25].

Myocardial biopsy reveals nonspecific findings with interstitial fibrosis and cellular hypertrophy like in other forms of cardiomyopathy [26].

12. Treatment

The cornerstone in this reversible cardiomyopathy is normalization of the heart rate either by medication, electrical cardioversion or catheter ablation. This results in decrease in the LV dimensions and increase in the LV ejection fraction [27, 28].

Antiarrhythmic drugs that can be used in patients, both pediatric and adults with tachycardia-induced cardiomyopathy, are the commonly used drugs in the Vaughan Williams classification: Ia, IB, Ic, II and III (both sotalol and amiodarone) as well as combinations. In the study of Moore et al. on pediatric population, most of the patients had amiodarone, beta-blockers or sotalol as treatment followed by Ic, Ia and lastly Ib. Ninety-two percent of patients treated with amiodarone had a positive response to this drug [29].

The catheter ablation technique depends on the principal mechanism of the arrhythmia: abnormal automaticity, triggered activity or reentry. Inappropriate sinus tachycardia is caused by enhanced normal automaticity, and ablation is performed in the region of the sinus node. Focal atrial tachycardia may be due to automaticity, triggered activity or microreentrant mechanism, and ablation is performed at the level of earliest atrial activation site. Typical atrial flutter has a macroreentrant circuit, where ablation is achieved at the level of cavo-tricuspid isthmus. Even though the mechanism of atrial fibrillation is still debated among electrophysiologists, drivers located at the level of pulmonary veins and rotors inside the left atrium are important in initiation and maintenance of the arrhythmia. Ablation for paroxysmal atrial fibrillation consists in pulmonary vein isolation (PVI) and for persistent atrial fibrillation PVI plus substrate modification. Atrioventricular nodal reentrant tachycardia is caused by a reentrant mechanism. The presence of two pathways within the AV node, slow pathway and fast pathway, makes the arrhythmia possible. Under normal condition, ablation is performed at the level of the slow pathway. Atrioventricular reentrant tachycardia mediated by an accessory pathway has also a macroreentrant mechanism. The circuit involves an accessory pathway that is usually ablated during the procedure.

In the absence of a structural heart disease, most ventricular tachycardias have an automatic mechanism or given by triggered activity. For outflow tract tachycardias, ablation is performed at the level of earliest ventricular activation site. Fascicular ventricular tachycardias are accepted to have a macroreentrant mechanism involving slow response fibers of the Purkinje network. Ablation is usually performed at this level or at the fascicular level (left postero-inferior or left antero-superior). Ventricular tachycardia in patients with old myocardial infarction, nonischemic cardiomyopathy or ventricular dysplasia has a reentry mechanism, but usually they are not responsible for tachycardia-induced cardiomyopathy.

http://dx.doi.org/10.5772/66515

We propose the following algorithm of treatment in patients suspected of tachycardia-induced cardiomyopathy: antiarrhythmic drugs should be started with the aim of normalization of the heart rate; in function of the arrhythmia and associated morbidities, beta-blockers can be initiated, than escalated to class IC (propafenone or flecainide) in case of no response in heart rate reduction. Amiodarone should be the last antiarrhythmic drug to be tested because of its side effects. In case of response to amiodarone with normalization of the heart rate and ejection fraction, a diagnosis of tachycardia-induced cardiomyopathy can be made and catheter ablation should be proposed. Catheter ablation aims to stop the long-term treatment with amiodarone.

13. Clinical case reports

13.1. Case report 1: PVCs >30,000/24 h

A 19-year-old male patient with >30% PVCs on 24 h was hospitalized for catheter ablation. Echocardiography confirmed tachycardia-induced cardiomyopathy with an EF of 35% (**Figure 1**). Cardiac MRI showed an EF of 37% with no sign of myocarditis or fibrosis. After ablation of monomorphic PVCs from the right ventricle (**Figure 2**), LV systolic function normalized with decrease in the dimensions of the heart chambers. At 3-month follow-up, the ejection fraction increased to 55%.

13.2. Case report 2: antidromic tachycardia

A 26-year-old male patient presented episodes of wide QRS tachycardia with depressed ejection fraction of 40% and a dilated left ventricle (**Figure 3**). His resting ECG showed short PR interval and presence of the delta wave (**Figure 4**). The abnormal activation of the left ventricle with intraventricular dissynchronism led to dilated cardiomyopathy. Beta-blockers were ineffective in controlling tachycardia, and catheter ablation was proposed. At 4-week follow-up after ablation, left ventricular function recovered with normalization of the end-systolic and end-diastolic LV diameters.

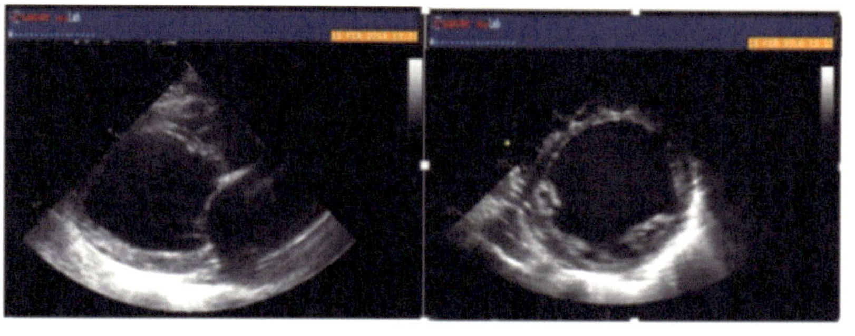

Figure 1. Bi-dimensional echocardiography apical view and parasternal short axis in a 19-year-old dilated left ventricle 63/54 with depressed ejection fraction of 35% in a patient with PVC-induced cardiomyopathy.

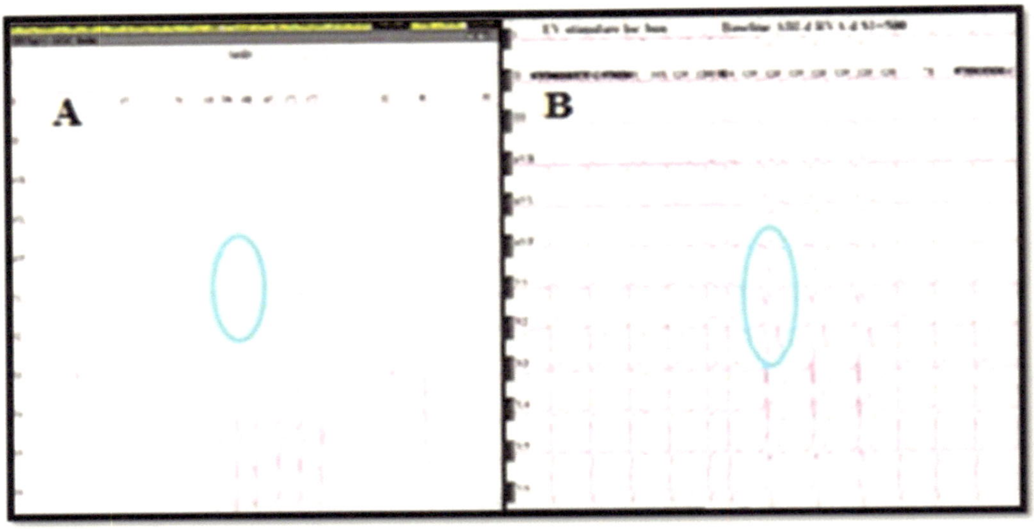

Figure 2. Pacemap inside the right ventricle to identify the origin of PVCs. (A) poor correlation pacemap-clinical PVC; (B) good correlation 12/12 pacemap-clinical PVC. At this spot, RF ablation determined complete resolution of PVCs with no recurrence. Holter ECG identified 0 ExV/24 h.

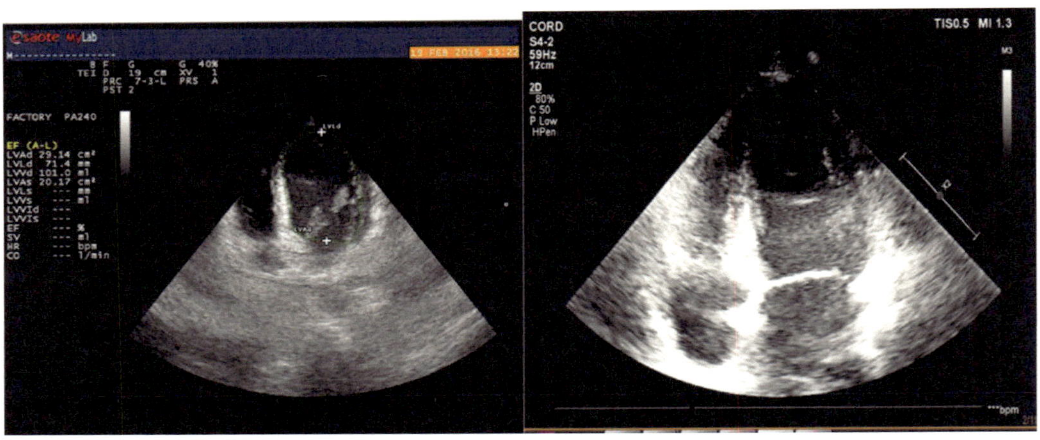

Figure 3. Echocardiography apical view before and after ablation of a left lateral accessory pathway with frequent episodes of antidromic tachycardia.

13.3. Case report 3: 2:1 atrial flutter

A 52-year-old male patient presented to the cardiology department with dyspnea and leg edema. His heart rate was 150 bpm (**Figure 5**), and blood pressure was 110/50 mmHg. Echocardiography revealed depressed ejection fraction of 35% with dilated left ventricle 60/50 and mitral regurgitation grade 2. Antiarrhythmic drug was ineffective in reducing arrhythmia with persistence of high rates 150 bpm after amiodarone, metoprolol and digoxin. He was

http://dx.doi.org/10.5772/66515

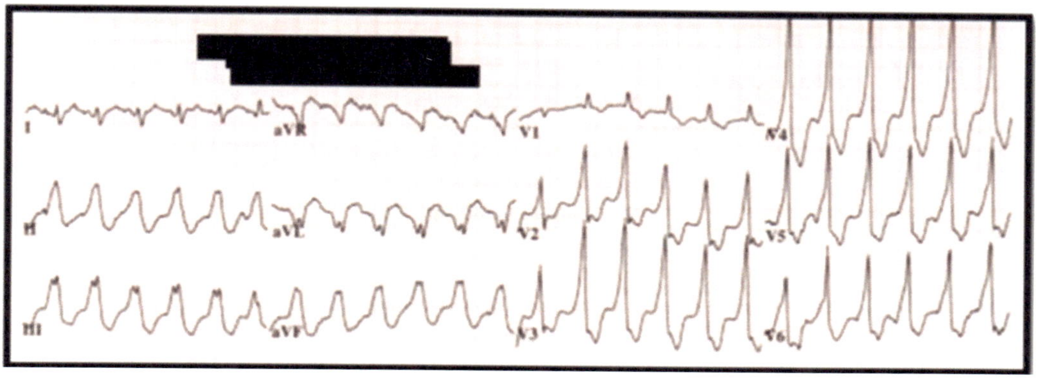

Figure 4. Twelve-lead ECG during antidromic tachycardia: wide QRS tachycardia 160/min with positive concordance in the precordial leads and negative QRS in lead I and aVL suggesting left lateral accessory pathway.

transferred in our department, and after ablation of the tricuspid isthmus sinus, rhythm was obtained. At 1-month follow-up, ejection fraction normalized >50% with left ventricular diameters of 45/25 and decrease in mitral regurgitation to grade 1 (**Figure 6**).

13.4. Case report 4: persistent atrial fibrillation

A 63-year-old male patient presented to our cardiology department an episode of persistent atrial fibrillation and heart failure. At physical examination, we noticed a heart rate of 120 bpm (**Figure 7**), arrhythmic, with systolic murmur in the left ventricular area, a blood pressure of 140/80 mmHg and signs of right heart failure: bilateral edema and hepatomegaly.

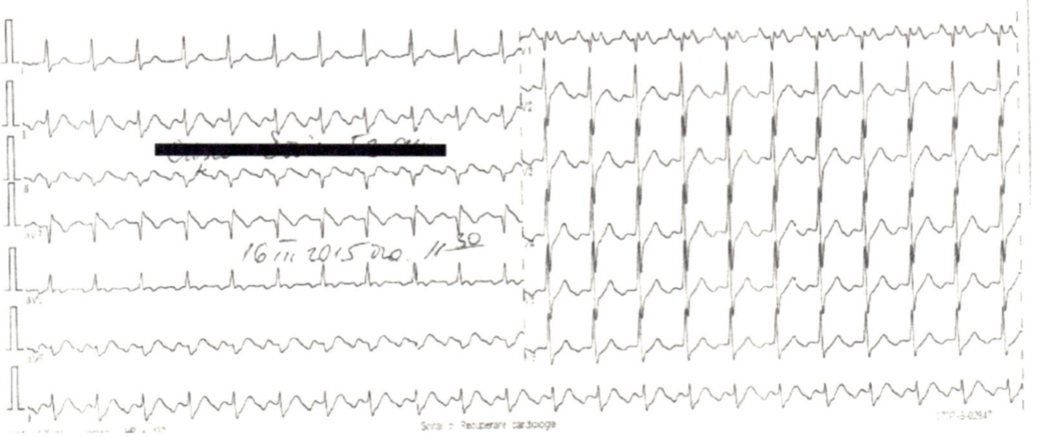

Figure 5. Twelve-lead ECG during 2:1 atrial flutter in a 52-year-old male patient with tachycardiomyopathy. F waves are negative in inferior leads: D2, D3 and aVF and positive in lead V1.

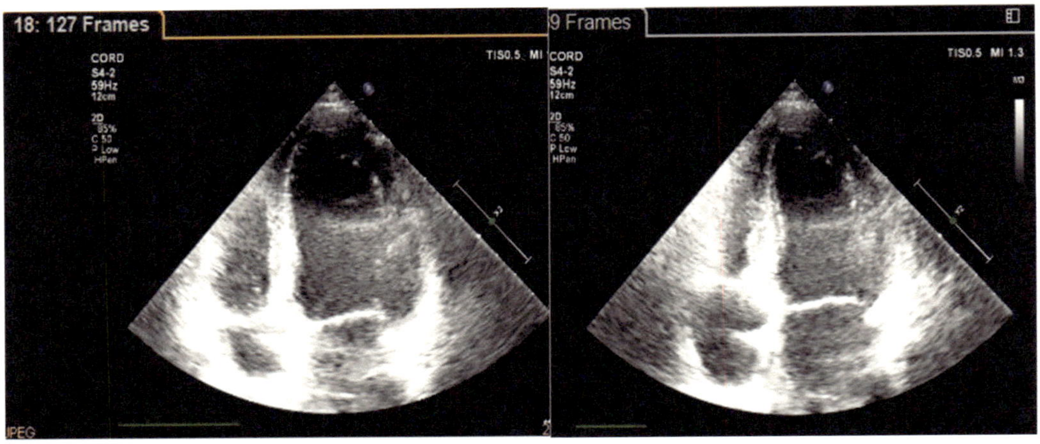

Figure 6. Echocardiography apical view before and after ablation of the cavo-tricuspid isthmus in a patient with dilated cardiomyopathy due to 2:1 typical atrial flutter.

Ejection fraction was 30% with mild dilatation of the left ventricle 65/55, mitral regurgitation grade II, left atrial dilation 53 mm and high pulmonary pressure 60 mmHg (**Figure 8**). Lab tests showed normal CBC, effective anticoagulation with an INR of 3.8, LDL = 53 mg% and triglycerides = 65 mg%, normal ASAT = 15 and normal ALAT = 12 mg%. Chest X-ray showed increased cardio-thoracic index (**Figure 9**).

After isolation of the left pulmonary veins (**Figure 10**), sinus rhythm was obtained. No pulmonary vein potentials were observed at the level of the right pulmonary veins (**Figure 11**). No

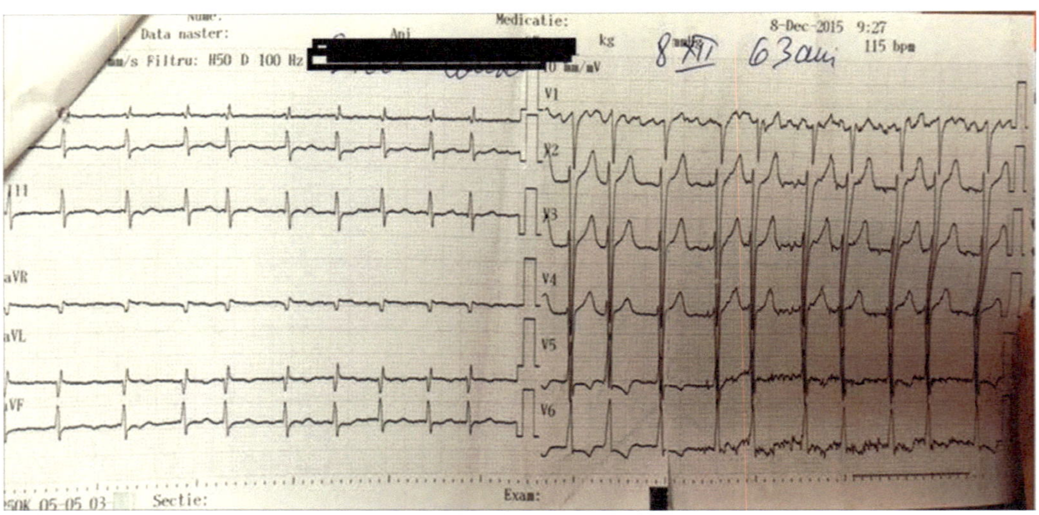

Figure 7. Twelve-lead ECG during atrial fibrillation in a 63-year-old male patient with tachycardiomyopathy. The amplitude of the f waves in lead V1 is in favor of a recent onset of atrial fibrillation.

http://dx.doi.org/10.5772/66515

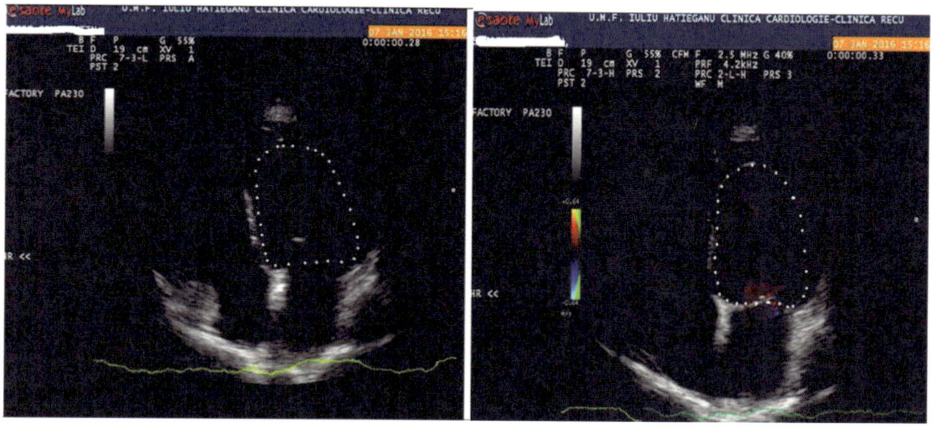

Figure 8. Echocardiography apical view before isolation of the pulmonary veins showing dilated left ventricle 65/55 mm with depressed ejection fraction of 30%, mitral regurgitation grade 2 and a dilated left atrium. Images after ablation at 3-month follow-up are not available.

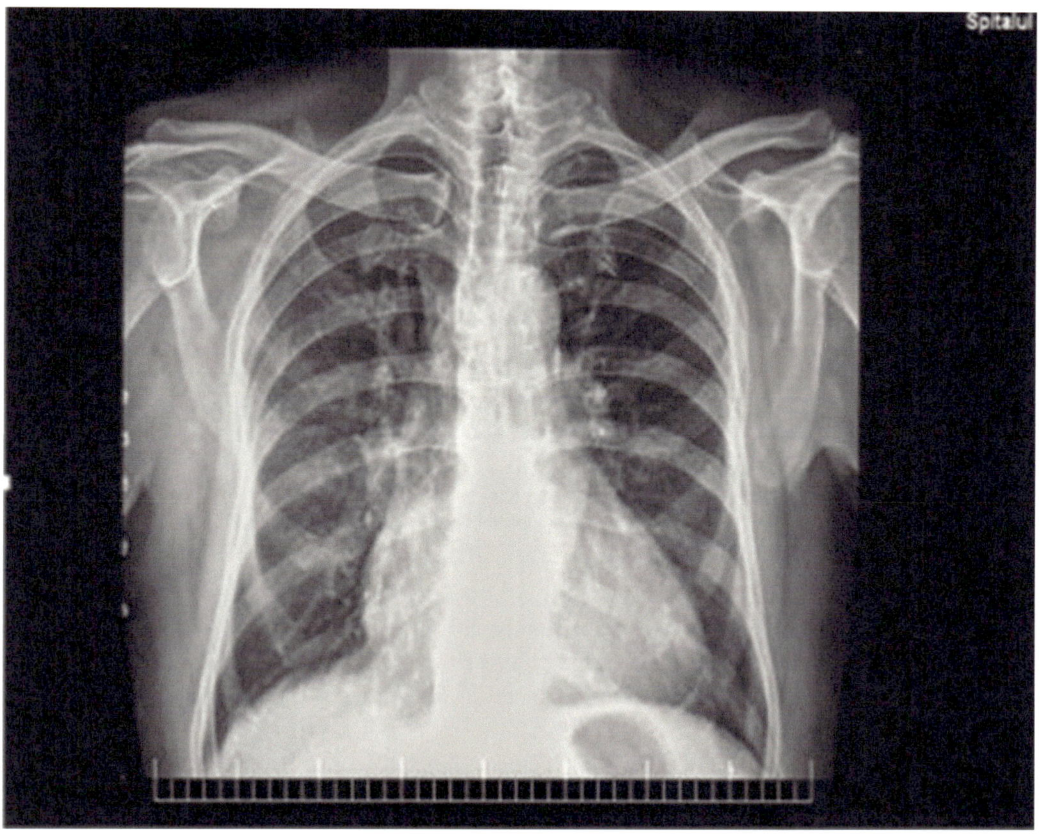

Figure 9. Chest X-ray AP view before ablation showing increased cardio-thoracic index.

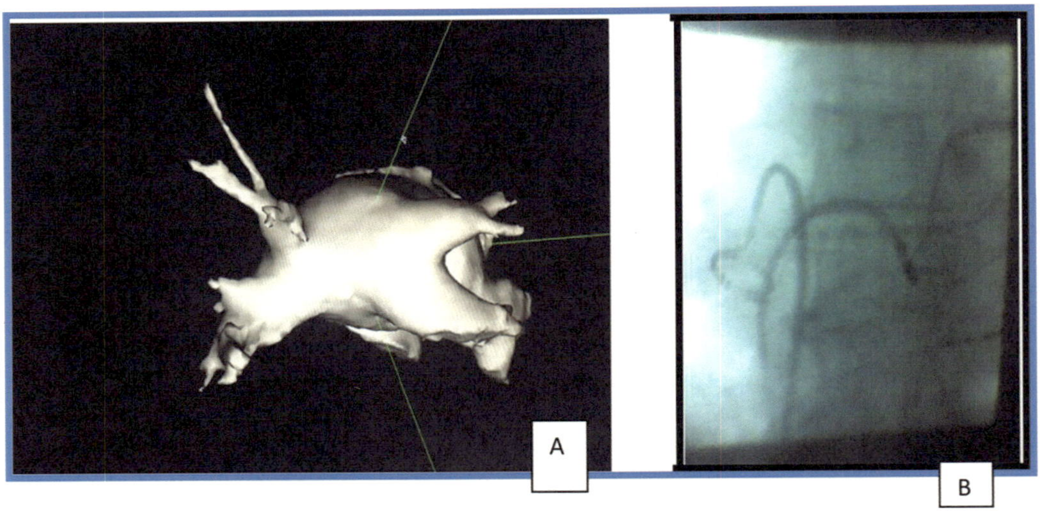

Figure 10. (A) Computed tomography with contrast shows four pulmonary veins: two on the left side and two on the right side and (B) X-ray during mapping of the right inferior pulmonary vein in the AP view. No PVPs were detected inside this vein.

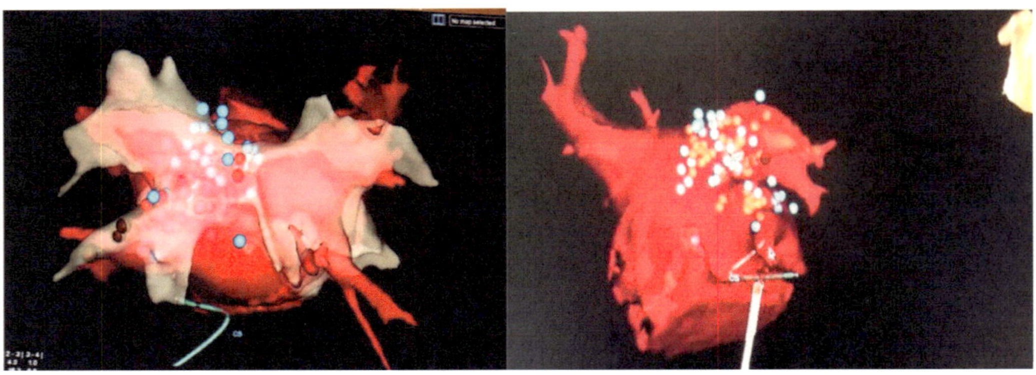

Figure 11. Images during the ablation procedure: only the left pulmonary veins were isolated because the right veins presented no PVP. On the left side: merge between scanner and NavX-Saint Jude mapped pulmonary veins.

left atrial substrate ablation was necessary for obtaining sinus rhythm. At 3-month follow-up, echocardiography in another cardiac department showed a normal ejection fraction of 50% with normal left ventricular diameters 52/26, mild dilatation of the left atrium 44 mm and mild mitral regurgitation.

13.5. Case report 5: RVOT PVCs and NSVT

A 28-year-old male patient was referred to us because of LV dysfunction, frequent PVCs and episodes of nonsustained VT.

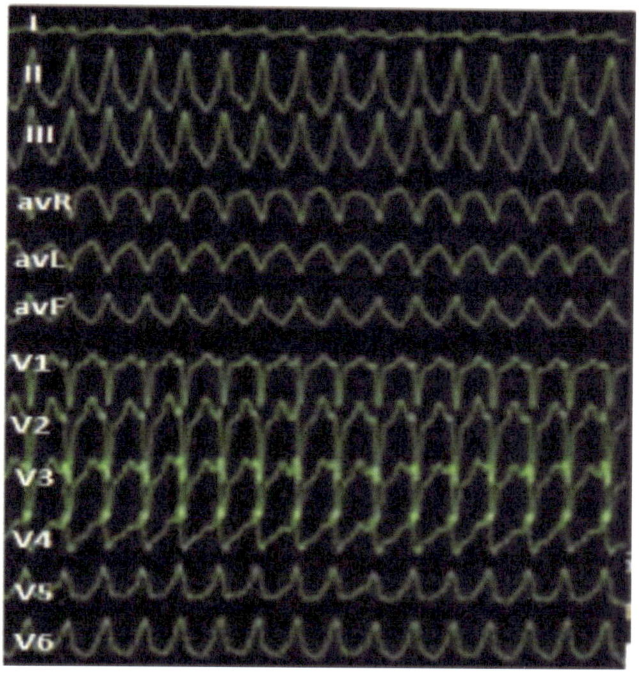

Figure 12. Nonsustained VT less than 30 s. The QRS morphology is compatible with RVOT origin: LBBB and inferior axis, transition in V4.

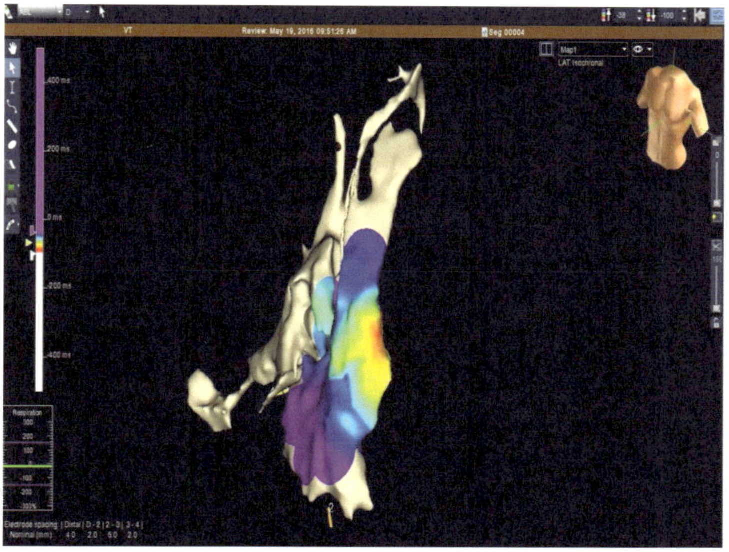

Figure 13. Three-dimensional activation mapping using the Navx-Saint Jude system. The earliest potential was recorded at the level of antero-septal RVOT (red color). RF ablation at this level stopped PVCs and rendered RVOT VT uninducible at stimulation after adrenalin infusion.

The patient's main complaint was palpitation with dyspnea during exertion. Echocardiography revealed an EF of 40% and mild dilation of the left ventricle. The QRS morphology was compatible with RVOT origin (**Figure 12**), and the high number of PVCs >35% on 24 h determined us to perform catheter ablation. After the ablation (**Figure 13**), no more PVC was present at follow-up and LV ejection fraction normalized with decrease in LV diameters to normal values.

14. Conclusion

Tachycardia-induced cardiomyopathy should be considered in all patients with depressed ejection fraction concomitant with a chronic tachyarrhythmia. It is a reversible cause of heart failure, and electrophysiological study and mapping should be considered early in the diagnosis and treatment algorithm of those patients. An aggressive approach by catheter ablation is important when this type of reversible cardiomyopathy is suspected.

As the clinical impact of ablation is substantial, we recommend it for the reversibility of both functional and structural changes induced by the tachyarrhythmia.

Author details

Cismaru Gabriel*, Lucian Muresan, Puiu Mihai, Radu Rosu, Gabriel Gusetu, Dana Pop and Dumitru Zdrenghea

*Address all correspondence to: gabi_cismaru@yahoo.com

Iuliu Hatieganu University od Medicine and Pharmacy, 5th Dept. of Internal Medicine, Cardiology Rehabilitation, Cluj-Rapoca, Romania

References

[1] Whipple GH, Sheffield LT, Woodman EG, Theophilis C, Friedman S. Reversible congestive heart failure due to chronic rapid stimulation of the normal heart. Proc N Engl Cardiovasc Soc 1962;20:39–40.

[2] Gentlesk PJ, Sauer WH, Gerstenfeld EP, Lin D, Dixit S, Zado E, et al. Reversal of left ventricular dysfunction following ablation of atrial fibrillation. J Cardiovasc Electrophysiol 2007;18:9–14.

[3] Medi C, Kalman JM, Haqqani H, et al. Tachycardia-mediated cardiomyopathy secondary to focal atrial tachycardia: long term outcome after catheter ablation. J Am Coll Cardiol 2009;53:1791–1797.

http://dx.doi.org/10.5772/66515

[4] Aguinaga L, Primo J, Anguera I, et al. Long-term follow-up in patients with the permanent form of functional reciprocating tachycardia treated with radiofrequency ablation. Pacing Clin Electrphysiol 1998;21:1073–1078.

[5] Wilkoff BL, Cook JR, Epstein AE, Greene HL, Hallstrom AP, Hsia H, Kutalek SP, et al. Dual-chamber pacing or ventricular backup pacing in patients with an implanted defibrillator: the Dual Chamber and VVI Implantable Defibrillator (DAVID) trial. JAMA 2002;288(24):3115–3123.

[6] Abraham WT, Fisher WG, Smith AL, Delrgio DB, Leon AR, Loh E, Kocovic DZ, et al. Cardiac resynchronization in chronic heart failure. N Engl J Med 2002;364(24):1845–1853.

[7] Tanaka R, Spinale FG, Crawford FA, Zille MR. Effect of chronic supraventricular tachycardia on left ventricular function and structure in newborn pigs. J Am Coll Cardiol 1992;20:1650–1660.

[8] Patel HJ, Pilla JJ, Polidori DJ, Pusca SV, Plappert TA, Sutton MS, Lankford EB, Acker MA. Ten weeks of rapid ventricular pacing creates a long-term model of left ventricular dysfunction. J Thorac Cardiovasc Surg 2000;119:834–841.

[9] Zellner JL, Spinale FG, Eble DM, Hewett KW, Crawford FA Jr. Alteration in myocite shape and basement attachment with tachycardia-induced heart failure. Circ Res 1991;69:590–600.

[10] O Brien PJ, Januzzo CD, Moe GW, Stoops TP, Armstrong PW. Rapid ventricular pacing of dogs to heart failure: biochemical and physiological studies. Can J Physiol Pharmacol 1990;68:34–39.

[11] Rosenbaum MB, Blanco HH, Elizari MV, Lazzari JO, Davidenko JM, Electronic modulation of the T wave and cardiac memory. Am. J Cardiol 1982;50:213–222.

[12] Freundlich J. Paroxysmal ventricular tachycardia. Am Heart J 1946;31:557.

[13] Dubbs AW, Parmet DH, Ventricular tachycardia stopped on the twenty-first day of giving quinidine sulfate intravenously. Am Heart J 1942;24:272.

[14] Campbell M. Inversion of T waves after long paroxysms of tachycardia. Br Heart J 1942;4:49.

[15] Han FT, Kiser R, Nixon JV, Wood MA, Ellenbogen KA. What is the time course of reversal of tachycardia-induced cardiomyopathy? Europace 2011;13:139–141.

[16] Chin A, Ntusi BM, Badri M. Clinical, electrocardiographic and echocardiographic characteristics of tachycardia-induced cardiomyopathy. Eur J Heart Fail Suppl 2010;9(Suppl. 1):5251.

[17] Nerheim P, Biger-Botkin S, Piracha L, Olhansky B. Heart failure and sudden cardiac death in patients with tachycardia-induced cardiomyopathy and recurrent tachycardia. Circulation 2004;110:247–252.

[18] Juneja R, Shah S, Naik N, Kothari SS, SaxenaA, Talwar KK. Management of cardiomyopathy resulting from incessant supraventricular tachycardia in infants and children. India Heart J 2002;54:176–180.

[19] Walker NL, Coobe SM, Birnie DH. Tachycardiomyopathy:a diagnosis not to be missed. Heart 2004;90:e7.

[20] Calo L, Sciarra L, Scioli R, Lamberti F, Loricchio ML, Pandozi C, Santini M. Recovery of cardiac function after ablation of atrial tachycardia arising from tricuspid annulus. Ital Heart J 2005;6:652–657.

[21] Salemi VM, Arteaga E, Mady C. Recovery of systolic and diastolic function after ablation of incessant supraventricular tachycardia. Eur J Heart Fail 2005;7:1177–1179.

[22] Rodrigues LM, Smees JL, Xie B. Improvement in left ventricular function by ablation of atrioventricular nodal conduction in selected patients with lone atrial fibrillation. Am J Cardiol 1993;72:1137–1141.

[23] Redfield MM, Kay GN, Jenkins LS, Mianulli M, Jensen DN, Ellenbogen KA. Tachycardia-related cardiomyopathy: a common cause of ventricular dysfunction in patients with atrial fibrillation referred for atrioventricular ablation. Mayo Clin Proc 200;75:790–7955.

[24] Hasdemir C, Yuksel A, Camil D et al. Late gadolinium enhancement CMR in patients with tachycardia-induced cardiomyopathy caused by idiopathic ventricular arrhythmia. Pacing Clin Electrophysiol 2012;35:465–470.

[25] Redfield MM, Aarhus LL, Wright RS, Burnett JC Jr. Cardiorenal and neurohormonal function in a canine model of early left ventricular dysfunction. Circulation 1993;87:2016–2022.

[26] Fenelon G, Wijns W, Andries E, Brugada P. Tachycardiomyopathy: mechanisms and clinical application. Pacing Clin Electrophysiol 1996;19:95–106.

[27] Packer DL, Bardy GH, Worley SJ, Smith MS, Cobb FR, Coleman RE, Gallagher JJ, German LD. Tachycardia-induced cardiomyopathy: a reversible form of left ventricular dysfunction. Am J Cardiol 1986;57:563–570.

[28] Kessler G, Roseblatt S, Friedman J, Kaplinsky E. Recurrent dilated cardiomyopathy reversed with cardioversion of atrial fibrillation. Am Heart J 1997;133:384–386.

[29] Alessandrini RS, McPherson DD, Kadish AH, Kane BJ, Goldberger JJ. Cardiac memory: a mechanical and electrical phenomenon. Am J Physiol 1997 Apr;272(4 Pt 2):H1952–9.

Section 4

Metabolic Impact on Systolic Heart Failure

Chapter 8

Impact of Thyroid Disease on Heart Failure

Adina Elena Stanciu, Adina Zamfir-Chiru-Anton,
Marcel Marian Stanciu and Dan Cristian Gheorghe

Additional information is available at the end of the chapter

http://dx.doi.org/10.5772/66283

Abstract

The modern vision concerning the physiological actions and pathological relevance of endocrine cardiac system is a very complex one. Decreased or increased action of thyroid hormone (hypo- or hyperthyroidism) on different cellular and molecular pathways in the heart plays an important role in the development and progression of myocardial remodelling and heart failure. Cardiovascular signs and symptoms that accompany both hyperthyroidism and hypothyroidism are presented, highlighting that correction of thyroid dysfunction most often reverses the abnormal cardiovascular hemodynamics.

Keywords: hyperthyroidism, hypothyroidism, heart failure, thyroid hormones, natriuretic peptides

1. Introduction

The modern vision concerning the physiological actions and pathological relevance of endocrine cardiac system is a very complex one. It is well-known that thyroid hormones and endocrine cardiac systems are strictly correlated in both physiological [1] and pathological conditions, especially in patients with cardiac diseases [2, 3]. Thyroid disease is the second most common endocrine disorder after diabetes mellitus, being present in 5–10% of the population. Current estimates suggest that the incidence of thyroid disease in adult female population is higher than in adult males, but with advancing age, especially beyond the eighth decade of life, the incidence in males rises to be equal to that of females [4]. Thyroid hormone has a homeostatic role on the cardiovascular system, especially in the presence of heart failure (HF). HF is a major public health issue, being currently diagnosed in approximately 23 million patients worldwide [5].

Many studies have recently confirmed that persistent subclinical thyroid dysfunction is associated with the development of HF by changes in cardiac structure and function [6, 7]. The term subclinical thyroid disease is used to define the state having an abnormal serum thyroid-stimulating hormone (TSH) concentration (below or above the statistically defined lower or upper limit of the reference range: 0.45–4.50 mIU/L) in the presence of normal serum thyroid hormones concentrations (free thyroxine and triiodothyronine within their reference ranges). Subclinical thyroid disease may progress to overt thyroid disease. Overt thyroid dysfunction is defined by an abnormality of both the TSH and thyroid hormones. Untreated overt hyperthyroidism and hypothyroidism have been reported to be common causes of HF [8].

Unfortunately, the impact of thyroid disease on HF and, implicitly, the full potential of the therapeutic use of thyroid hormones in treating and/or preventing HF, has not been adequately studied. This chapter addresses the effects of thyroid hormones on cardiac function and the clinical consequences of thyroid dysfunction.

2. Cellular and molecular mechanisms underlying the effects of thyroid hormones on the cardiovascular system

The hypothalamic-pituitary-thyroid axis is responsible for the regulation of thyroid metabolism involving the following steps: (step 1) hypothalamus produces thyrotropin-releasing hormone (TRH), needed to monitor the thyroid hormone concentrations; (step 2) TRH stimulates the pituitary to produce TSH; (step 3) under the action of TSH, thyroid gland secretes 85–90% thyroxine (T4) and 10–15% triiodothyronine (T3), the primary circulating thyroid hormones; (step 4) T4 is converted to T3 by the deiodinase system (D1–D3) in the liver, kidney, and skeletal muscle; (step 5) thyroxine binding globulin (TBG) is responsible for carrying T4 and T3 to the tissues.

Maintenance of thyroid hormone homeostasis is required for proper cardiovascular function [9]. Actually, an altered thyroid hormone metabolism leads to cardiac parameters changes by acting on some molecular pathways involved in cardiac hypertrophy and HF progression. Thyroid hormone may act directly on transcription on specific and nonspecific cardiac genes that include α and β myosin heavy chain (MHC-α and MHC-β, respectively), sarcoplasmic reticulum Ca^{2+}-ATPase (SERCA), atrial natriuretic peptide, sodium-potassium adenosine triphosphatase (Na-K-ATPase), β-adrenergic receptor and cardiac troponin I (genomic effect) [10–12], or on plasma membrane, sarcoplasmic reticulum (a specialized type of smooth endoplasmic reticulum that regulates the calcium ion concentration in the cytoplasm of striated muscle cells) and mitochondria (nongenomic effect) [13].

Many invasive and noninvasive measurements have shown that T3 plays an important role in modulating cardiac function [14]. T3 is the active form of thyroid hormone in the heart, because no significant myocyte intracellular deiodinase activity takes place at heart level. In fact, there is no experimental study to prove the conversion of T4 to T3 in cardiomyocytes. Due to their lipophilic nature, T3 and T4 can easily diffuse through the cytoplasmic membrane of cardiomyocytes. Lipophilic T3 enters the nucleus and binds to inactive nuclear thyroid hormone

http://dx.doi.org/10.5772/66283

receptors, which are encoded by the c-erbA proto-oncogene families. Further, the complex recognizes one of the several DNA consensus sequences and the thyroid response elements, located in the enhancer region of target genes [15]. The subsequent binding of the T3-receptor complexes to DNA regulates the expression of genes, encoding for structural and functional cardiac proteins (regulating calcium cycling in the cardiac myocyte) [16]. Thus, T3 modulates heart rate, cardiac contractility and arterial peripheral resistance, being essential to preserve both cardiac morphology and performance in adult life. In these circumstances, it is easy to understand why an altered thyroid status in patients with cardiovascular disorders could modify cardiac gene expression and contribute to impaired cardiac function.

A decrease in serum T3 needs to be analysed very carefully, because there are two possible causes: (i) low levels of T3 associated with low levels of T4 and high levels of TSH suggest a dysfunction of the thyroid gland itself (hypothyroidism), most often caused by an autoimmune disease (Hashimoto's thyroiditis) and/or iodine deficiency; (ii) low levels of T3 or free T3 (FT3) with normal T4 and low or normal TSH suggest a dysfunction which is unrelated to thyroid gland. This particular pattern has three names as follows: euthyroid sick syndrome, non-thyroidal illness syndrome, or low T3 syndrome.

The exact cause of low T3 syndrome is not known, but it is assumed that it occurs as a result of modified expression of the deiodinases (reduced enzyme activity of 5-monodeiodinase responsible for converting T4 into T3 in peripheral tissues) [17], modified entry of thyroid hormone into tissue (damage membrane) [18], or altered signalling due to changes in thyroid hormone receptors. Clinical and experimental evidence have shown that low T3 syndrome has been found in about 30% of HF patients, being associated with HF New York Heart Association (NYHA) functional class III–IV [19]. Furthermore, low T3 syndrome is considered a strong prognostic predictor of death in patients with HF, contributing to the progressive deterioration of cardiac function and myocardial remodelling in HF [17]. This might be explained by the fact that HF develops as the result of the added stress of health conditions, and a single risk factor may be sufficient to cause this syndrome.

Risk factors	**Inflammatory markers**	**Cellular events**	**Cardiac events**
Thyroid dysfunction	IL-1 β, IL-6, IL-8,	Fibroblast proliferation	Cardiac failure
Diabetes	TNF-α, CRP	Collagen synthesis	
Viral infections		Matrix metalloproteinases activation	
High blood pressure		Mechanical stress	
Coronary artery disease		Cardiomyocyte hypertrophy	
Heart attack		Cardiomyocyte apoptosis/necrosis	
Congenital heart defects			
Heart arrhythmias			
Valvular heart disease			

Table 1. Risk factors and mechanisms that are involved in the development of heart failure.

Actually, pathophysiological phenomena behind HF involve a compensatory activation of hormonal, neurohumoral, immunological, and proinflammatory systems as can be seen from **Table 1**.

Thyroid dysfunction triggers an inflammatory cascade. The balance between T-helper type 1 (Th1) and type 2 (Th2) lymphocytes may determine the outcome of autoimmune thyroid diseases. According to cytokine profiles, both Th1 and Th2 response have been supposed to be involved in the pathogenesis of Hashimoto's thyroiditis (the most common cause of hypothyroidism) and Graves' disease (the most common cause of hyperthyroidism), but with deviation toward Th1 pattern in Hashimoto's thyroiditis and toward Th2 pattern in Graves' disease. Autoimmune thyroid diseases have serum antibodies reacting with thyroglobulin, thyroid peroxidase, or TSH receptor and these antibodies might be cytotoxic. High antibodies concentrations correlate with proinflammatory cytokines, including interleukin-6 (IL-6) and tumour necrosis factor-α (TNF-α), responsible for oxidative stress, thyroid damage, and the loss of thyroid function [20]. Furthermore, many studies have shown that proinflammatory cytokines (IL-6, IL-1β, and TNF-α) are cardiodepressant and play a pathogenic role in HF, contributing to cardiac remodelling, which is a progressive process (**Table 1**). Also, it is known that IL-6 is a hallmark of the acute phase of low T3 syndrome [21]. Inflammatory biomarker C-reactive protein (CRP) is mainly produced in response to IL-6 and plays many pathophysiological roles in the inflammatory process in HF, in direct relation to deterioration of NYHA functional class and cardiac performance. In patients with Hashimoto's thyroiditis, there was a positive correlation between TgAb and hs-CRP ($r = 0.55$, $P = 0.01$) [22], CRP being inversely correlated with T3 and T3 levels, inversely correlated to the presence and severity of HF [23].

Plasma concentration of natriuretic peptides, including B-type natriuretic peptide (BNP), particularly its amino-terminal fragment (NT-proBNP) and A-type natriuretic peptide (ANP), and especially its amino-terminal fragment (NT-proANP) or mid-regional fragment (MR-proANP), can be used as an initial diagnostic test of HF, especially in the non-acute setting when echocardiography is not immediately available [24]. NT-proBNP, NT-proANP, and MR-proANP have longer half-lives, are more stable and, consequently, are more reliable analytes of prolonged cardiac overload than are the biologically active peptides [25]. NT-proBNP is considered a prognostic determinant of HF progression, it levels paralleling the degree of left ventricular dysfunction [26]. High NT-proBNP concentrations predict cardiac-related mortality in HF patients.

Recent attention has been drawn to the relation of thyroid hormone, inflammatory biomarkers, such as IL-6 and CRP, and natriuretic peptides. Many authors studied natriuretic peptides levels in different thyroid function states and found that their serum levels were strongly affected by thyroid function. Generally, natriuretic peptides are elevated in overt and subclinical hyperthyroidism and reduced in overt and subclinical hypothyroidism. Thus, Christ-Crain et al. [27] have found statistically significant higher serum NT-proBNP and proANP concentration in hyperthyroid patients compared to hypothyroid and euthyroid subjects. Kato et al. [28] measured ANP and BNP levels in 130 patients with thyrotoxicosis and correlated them with HF severity and thyroid function. The levels of BNP and ANP were elevated in thyrotoxic patients. After therapy, when euthyroidism was established, a normalization of their levels has

http://dx.doi.org/10.5772/66283

been noted. The authors concluded that the measurement of serum BNP levels in thyrotoxic patients is useful for monitoring cardiovascular conditions of HF. Pakula et al. [29] assessed echocardiographically diameters of cardiac cavities, left ventricular mass, left ventricular ejection fraction, and NT-proBNP in 101 patients with thyroid dysfunction, free from any cardiovascular disease. They have shown that hyperthyroidism, in both its clinical and subclinical forms, results in a significant increase in NT-proBNP serum levels, their results being in line to those obtained by Christ-Crain et al. [27]. Moreover, they noted that despite normalization of plasma levels of TSH, the treatment with levothyroxine (L-T4) did not restore a hyperthyroidism-induced increase in plasma NT-proBNP levels. These findings are in accordance with Stanciu et al. [30], who investigated the effects of short-term overt hypothyroidism and exogenous subclinical hyperthyroidism on NT-proBNP and NT-proANP, in patients with differentiated thyroid cancer treated with radioactive iodine (^{131}I—RAI). As illustrated in **Figures 1** and **2**, serum levels of NT-proBNP and NT-proANP were significantly higher in subclinical hyperthyroidism (t2) than in overt hypothyroidism (t1) (6185 ng/L, IQR: 1689–8778 ng/L vs. 21.6 ng/L, IQR: 13.9–203 ng/L and 674 ng/L, IQR: 529–858 ng/L vs. 309 ng/L, IQR: 23.7–580 ng/L, respectively, $P < 0.001$). The authors have found that FT3 positively regulates NT-proANP production from cardiac myocytes, NT-proANP more accurately reflecting direct thyroid hormone effects, than NT-proBNP. Stanciu et al. concluded that short-term acute hypothyroidism, due to L-T4 withdrawal, and subclinical hyperthyroidism, due to suppressive doses of L-T4, induce deleterious effects on natriuretic peptides profiles during RAI therapy.

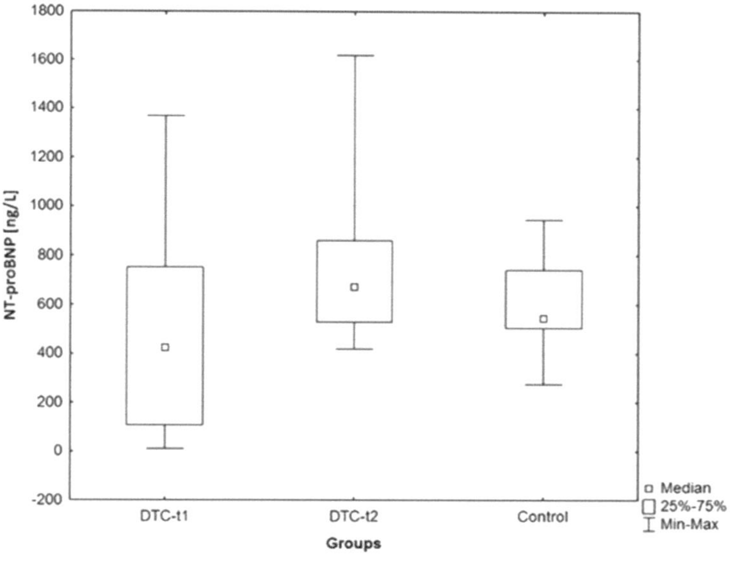

Figure 1. Median NT-proBNP levels in patients with differentiated thyroid cancer (DTC) compared with healthy euthyroid controls. DTC-t1: short-term overt hypothyroidism after levothyroxine withdrawal; DTC-t2: subclinical hyperthyroidism during suppressive levothyroxine therapy ($P < 0.001$ vs. DTC and healthy controls; $P < 0.001$ vs. DTC-t1 and DTC-t2).

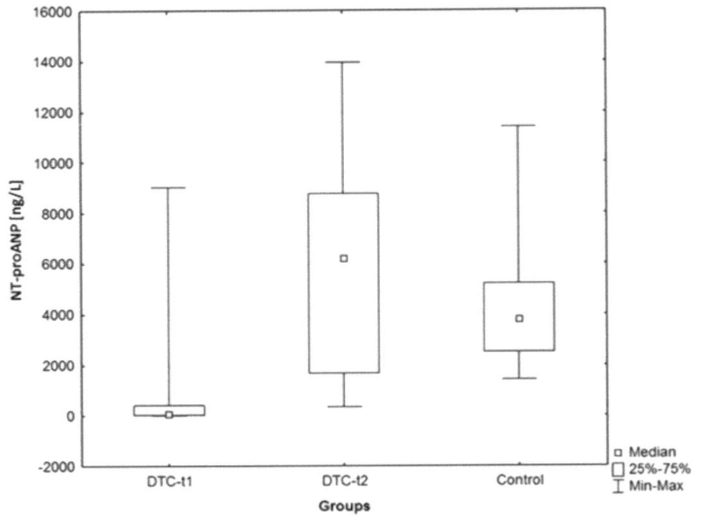

Figure 2. Median NT-proANP levels in patients with differentiated thyroid cancer (DTC) compared with healthy euthyroid controls. DTC-t1: short-term overt hypothyroidism after levothyroxine withdrawal; DTC-t2: subclinical hyperthyroidism during suppressive levothyroxine therapy ($P < 0.001$ vs. DTC and healthy controls; $P < 0.001$ vs. DTC-t1 and DTC-t2).

Brozaitiene et al. [31] studied the relationship and prognostic impact of thyroid hormones, inflammatory biomarkers, and NT-proBNP on long-term outcomes in coronary artery disease (CAD) patients with HF. Multivariate linear regression models, adjusted for age, gender, and body mass index, revealed that (ln) NT-proBNP was associated with hs-CRP ($\beta = 0.59$, $P < 0.001$), (ln) IL-6 ($\beta = 0.254$, $P < 0.001$), free thyroxine (FT4) ($\beta = 0.100$, $P = 0.011$), and T4 ($\beta = 0.112$, $P = 0.019$). Their results showed that thyroid hormones (i.e. FT4 level and FT3/FT4 ratio) together with NT-proBNP level may be valuable and simple predictors of long-term outcomes of CAD patients after experiencing acute coronary syndrome.

The question is: is this due to a compensatory mechanism, secondary to the thyroid hormone changes, or is it due to a direct action of thyroid hormone on the secretion of natriuretic peptides? The presented data have shown that natriuretic peptides are directly stimulated and regulated by thyroid hormones and immunological factors. Thyroid dysfunction triggers proinflammatory cytokines, known as stimulators of NT-proANP and NT-proBNP release. All of these leads to the idea that the thyrometabolic state must be taken into account when NT-proBNP or NT-proANP are assessed as markers of HF.

3. Impact of hyperthyroidism on heart failure

Endogenous hyperthyroidism (overproduction of thyroid hormone) and exogenous hyperthyroidism (ingestion of excessive amounts of thyroid hormone, i.e. suppressive doses of L-T4 to treat thyroid cancer) are associated with palpitations, tachycardia, exercise intolerance, dyspnea on exertion and increased heart rate. Patients with overt and subclinical hyperthyroidism are at increased risk of atrial arrhythmias and HF, because long-term exposure to thyroid hormone excess exerts unfavourable effects on cardiac morphology and function by increasing left ventricular mass, arterial stiffness, and left atrial size [32]. More than that, autoimmune hyperthyroidism (Graves' disease) has been frequently linked to autoimmune cardiovascular involvement (pulmonary arterial hypertension, myxomatous cardiac valve disease, and autoimmune cardiomyopathy). The effects of thyroid hormones on the heart and peripheral vasculature include decreased systemic vascular resistance (SVR) and diastolic blood pressure and increased resting heart rate, left ventricular contractility and pulmonary arterial pressure, as can be seen from **Table 2**. In overt hyperthyroidism, these combined effects increase cardiac output by 50–300% more than in normal subjects [33], resulting in right ventricular failure, as a consequence of immune-mediated endothelial damage [34]. Also, in patients with overt hyperthyroidism, a high prevalence of left ventricular hypertrophy and an increase in the contractility of the left ventricle and ejection fraction have been reported [34].

Variables	Hyperthyroidism	Hypothyroidism
Thyroid hormones	↑	↓
Oxidative metabolism	↑	↓
Natriuretic peptides	↑	↓
Lipids and lipoproteins	↓	↑
Heart rate	↑	↓
Systemic vascular resistance	↓	↑
Cardiac output	↑	↓
Cardiac contractility	↑	↓

Note: ↑, increased; ↓, decreased.

Table 2. Cardiovascular effects of thyroid dysfunction.

Subclinical hyperthyroidism can contribute to HF by increasing of heart rate and left ventricular mass, by worsening diastolic function and by predisposing to atrial fibrillation (AF) [35]. AF occurs in 10–25% of patients with hyperthyroidism (subclinical hyperthyroidism: RR = 1.31; 95% CI: 1.19–1.44 and overt hyperthyroidism RR = 1.42; 95% CI: 1.22–1.63) [36]. Actually, hyperthyroidism alters cardiac ion channel expression and function, increases heart rate and shortens atrial effective refractory period (ERP). The main cellular mechanisms of atrial contractile dysfunction are downregulation of the Ca^{2+} inward current and impaired release of Ca^{2+}. In fact, downregulation of the L-type Ca^{2+} inward current and upregulation of inward rectifier K^+ currents lead to shortening of action potential duration and atrial EPR, providing a substrate for AF. High levels of thyroid hormones can increase automaticity and enhance triggered activity in cardiomyocytes from pulmonary veins, resulting in atrial tachyarrhythmias.

In the last few years, many authors have attempted to show that exogenous subclinical hyperthyroidism, due to suppressive doses of L-T4, exerts many significant effects on the cardiovascular system, resulting in cardiovascular dysfunction [34–39]. A population-based prospective study was conducted in Denmark [38]. A total of 609 subjects from general practice, aged 50 years or above, with normal left ventricular function, were examined during a median of 5 years of follow-up. The incidence of stroke was increased among subjects with subclinical hyperthyroidism, HR = 3.39 (95% CI: 1.15–10.00, $P = 0.027$) after adjusting for sex, age, and AF. The authors concluded that subclinical hyperthyroidism seems to be a risk factor of developing major cardiovascular events, especially stroke in older adults from the general population with normal left ventricular function.

Collet et al. [39] performed another large analysis of prospective cohort studies. Individual data on 52,674 participants were pooled from 10 cohorts. Coronary heart disease events were analysed in 22,437 participants from 6 cohorts with available data, and the incidence of AF was analysed in 8711 participants from 5 cohorts. The study results showed that endogenous subclinical hyperthyroidism is associated with an increased risk of coronary heart disease mortality, and incident AF, with highest risks of coronary heart disease mortality, AF and HF when TSH level is lower than 0.10 mIU/L.

However, all these alterations may be reversible or may improve with the achievement of euthyroidism, because an excess of thyroid hormone does not induce cardiac fibrosis. Actually, the goal of thyroid dysfunction treatment is to restore the euthyroid state and avoid potential side effects.

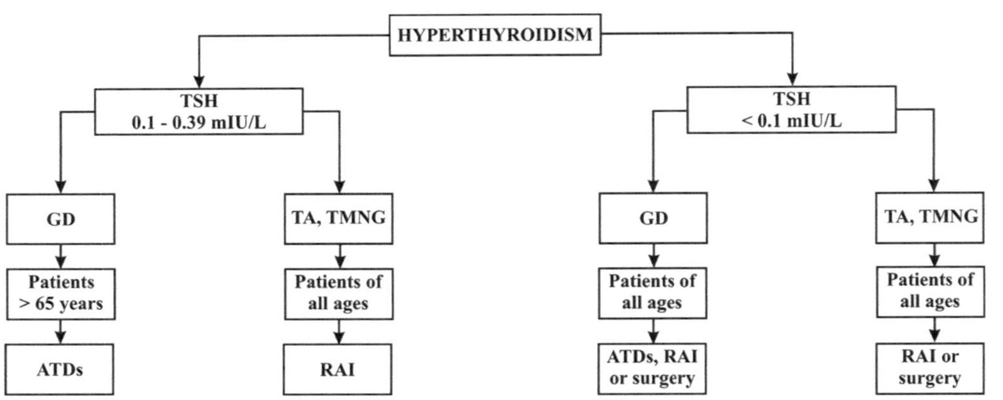

Figure 3. Algorithm for the treatment of hyperthyroidism in patients with atrial fibrillation and/or heart failure. TSH: thyroid-stimulating hormone; GD: Graves' disease; TA: toxic adenoma; TMNG: toxic multinodular goitre; ATDs: anti-thyroid drugs; RAI: radioactive iodine.

An algorithm for the treatment of hyperthyroidism in patients with AF and/or HF is presented in **Figure 3**. The first-line therapy in patients older than 65 years of age with hyperthyroidism, due to Graves' disease, should be the treatment with anti-thyroid drugs (carbimazole or its metabolite methimazole) in order to obtain spontaneous conversion to sinus rhythm. Ablative therapy (surgery or RAI) is the best treatment option in patients with hyperthyroidism, due to toxic adenoma (TA) or toxic multinodular goitre (TMNG), and concomitant heart disease, as can be seen in **Figure 3**. RAI therapy is much safer than it sounds and has no associated complications [40]. Also, ablative therapy may be recommended for patients with Graves' disease if the treatment with anti-thyroid drugs fails [32]. Nevertheless, HF may become irreversible in some cases of autoimmune hyperthyroid cardiomyopathy with a low ejection fraction [41].

4. Impact of hypothyroidism on heart failure

As shown in **Table 2**, in hypothyroidism, cardiovascular effects are diametrically opposed to hyperthyroidism and cardiac output declines by 30–50% [33]. Hypothyroidism is associated with bradycardia, reduced pulse pressure, cold intolerance, mild diastolic hypertension, and fatigue.

Significant changes in cardiac structure and function have been reported in patients with hypothyroidism, with a severity depending on the degree and length of thyroid hormone deficiency [42–48]. Overt hypothyroidism affects approximately 3% of the adult female population. Overt and subclinical hypothyroidism results in an increased SVR with a reduced cardiac output, a reduction in heart rate, an increased prevalence of hypertension, changes in cardiac natriuretic hormones, changes in lipid profile, accelerated atherosclerosis, damage of the physical and intellectual capacities, and an impaired quality of life. Hypothyroidism is a risk factor of HF in the general population. Several similarities have been observed between acute hypothyroidism and HF, including: decreased cardiac output; decreased cardiac contractility and an altered gene expression profile (alteration in myosin heavy chain isoform expression and alterations in the activity of the sarcoplasmic reticulum Ca^{2+} pump that are induced by its interactions with phospholamban, a reversible inhibitor). In most cases, these changes are the result of reduced T3 level (<3.1 pmol/L), the physiological T3 therapy improving cardiac function.

A systematic review and meta-analysis to clarify the association of hypothyroidism and all-cause mortality, as well as cardiac death and/or hospitalization in patients with HF, was conducted by Ning et al. [49]. They included 13 articles that reported relative risks estimates and 95% confidence intervals for hypothyroidism with outcomes in patients with HF. The authors found hypothyroidism associated with increased all-cause mortality as well as cardiac death and/or hospitalization in patients with HF.

Multiple cardiac effects of hypothyroidism have been reviewed by Biondi and Cooper [50]. Left ventricular diastolic dysfunction was found at rest and exercise in subclinical hyperthyroidism by Doppler echocardiography and radionuclide ventriculography. The isovolumetric relaxation time is prolonged and filling rate is impaired compared with controls. Actually, the most common cardiac abnormality in subclinical hypothyroidism is left ventricular diastolic dysfunction, characterized by slowed myocardial relaxation, and impaired ventricular filling. Impaired left ventricular systolic function is not commonly reported, but was identified using more sensitive techniques [50]. Cardiac effects due to subclinical hypothyroidism are less serious but somewhat similar to those seen in overt hypothyroidism, suggesting a continuum in the impact of thyroid hormone on the heart. Overt hypothyroidism is usually associated with grade I diastolic dysfunction, but grade II diastolic dysfunction, called "pseudonormal filling dynamics", can also be found [51].

There are also data showing that hypothyroidism results in an increased AF susceptibility (HR = 1.23; 95% CI: 0.77–1.97) [36], quite similar to hyperthyroidism, but affecting other atrial electrophysiological parameters than hyperthyroidism. Hypothyroidism alters cardiac ion channel expression and function, decreases heart rate, and prolongs sinus node recovery time and atrial ERP. In hypothyroid patients, increased atrial interstitial collagen may contribute to longer atrial ERP and lead to increased conduction heterogeneity, thus favouring re-entry formation and AF vulnerability. On the other hand, ion channel remodelling and dispersion may enhance AF arrhythmogenesis.

L-T4 replacement therapy reduces myocyte apoptosis and is able to improve cardiovascular performance and ventricular remodelling in hypothyroidism [52, 53]. It is important to recognize that normal cardiovascular hemodynamic restoration can take place without a significant increase in resting heart rate in the treatment of hypothyroidism. Treatment and management of subclinical and overt hypothyroidism should be tailored to each patient. L-T4 dose varies according to age, weight, severity, and duration of hypothyroidism and cardiac condition of the patient. Treatment of subclinical and overt hypothyroidism with appropriate doses of L-T4 has shown benefits in restoring of normal TSH values (after 6–12 months of substitution therapy). In hypothyroidism, systolic and diastolic functions (left ventricular predominantly) are affected. For patients with systolic and diastolic HF and in the elderly (>70 years), a small dose of L-T4 should be started, 25 or 50 mcg daily. The dose of L-T4 should be increased by 25 mcg/day every three to four weeks until a full replacement dosage is reached. This treatment should be individualized and permanently monitored, the aim being to reach a stable serum TSH around 1–5 mIU/L. A special attention should be given to the oldest old subjects (>80–85 years) with elevated serum TSH ≤ 10 mIU/L. These patients should be carefully followed with a wait-and-see strategy, generally avoiding hormonal treatment [54].

5. Perspectives and conclusions

Thyroid dysfunction is a common clinical problem that has key role in regulating the cardiovascular system and may contribute to the clinical course of CAD, HF, and arrhythmic events. Actually, interrelations between thyroid function and cardiovascular system are manifold. Changes in euthyroid status may induce cardiovascular abnormalities and various cardiovascular pathologies may alter thyroid function. Also, cardiac medication can unbalance or impair thyroid function. These things have to be taken into account in the assessment and treatment of cardiovascular disease. Thus, thyroid function tests are needed in patients receiving amiodarone and when thyroid dysfunction is considered a possible or concomitant cause of HF.

Secondary cardiovascular events require an early diagnosis to prevent complications and establish a therapeutic conduct, with restoration of euthyroid status. An echocardiogram is necessary to detect ventricular, valvular, and atrial disease. The use of Doppler echocardiography is mandatory to assess cardiac function, pulmonary pressure, valve disease, and pleural or pericardial effusion in symptomatic patients with thyroid dysfunction. It is desirable to use newer echocardiographic methods such as 3D echocardiography or speckle tracking echocardiography for a more accurate assessment of myocardial function, offering a comprehensive approach and a better assessment in the early stages of cardiac dysfunction in patients with impaired thyroid.

Many authors have reported that thyroid dysfunction correction spontaneously converts AF to sinus rhythm in up to two-thirds of patients [36]. Unfortunately, one-third of patients remain in AF despite euthyroid state restoration, radiofrequency (RF) catheter ablation being the only therapeutic option. Normalization of thyroid function prior to the RF ablation reduces the risk of recurrence. Also, recommendations for antithrombotic prophylaxis are the same as for patients without thyroid disease. If thyroid dysfunction persists (i.e. thyrotoxicosis), despite an appropriate treatment, administration of a β-blocker (i.e. β-blockers are useful in cases of thyroid storm) is recommended to control the rate of ventricular response. The β-blocker will be replaced by a non-dihydropyridine calcium channel antagonist (diltiazem or verapamil) if contraindications exist.

The management of thyroid dysfunction in patients who receive left ventricular assist device (LVAD) or cardiac transplantation has not been directly addressed by recent guidelines. Thyroid disease is not a contraindication to transplantation, but is a risk factor. That is why, restoration of the euthyroid state should be the first-step prior LVAD or cardiac transplantation. Unfortunately, drugs administration such as amiodarone and anti-coagulants presents a management dilemma.

In conclusion, correction of thyroid dysfunction should be the first procedure in patients with coexisting cardiac impairment, in order to improve cardiac hemodynamics [24]. Despite message currently taught, thyroid hormones are too dangerous to treat patients, in the last few years, clinical and experimental evidence suggests that thyroid may be a target for HF treatment, thyroid hormone therapy improving clinical outcomes in HF [55–59]. It has been proven that thyroid hormones have anti-apoptotic, anti–inflammatory, anti-fibrotic and anti-remodelling effects, promoting angiogenesis and regeneration [57]. L-T4, L-T3, or thyroid hormone analogue diiodothyropropionic acid (DITPA) have been tested in patients with HF, but unfortunately, the protocols used for thyroid hormones administration were much different, affecting the results. However, preliminary data suggest that thyroid hormone therapy in patients with HF is safe, the benefits being substantial. Further studies are necessary to confirm, highlight, and explore the full potential of the therapeutic use of thyroid hormones in treating and/or preventing HF.

Author details

Adina Elena Stanciu[1*], Adina Zamfir-Chiru-Anton[2], Marcel Marian Stanciu[3] and Dan Cristian Gheorghe[4]

*Address all correspondence to: adinaelenastanciu@yahoo.com

1 Department of Carcinogenesis and Molecular Biology, Institute of Oncology Bucharest, Bucharest, Romania

2 ENT Department, Grigore Alexandrescu Children's Emergency Hospital, Bucharest, Romania

3 Electrical Engineering Faculty, University Politehnica of Bucharest, Bucharest, Romania

4 ENT Department, Maria Sklodowska Curie Children's Emergency Hospital, Bucharest, Romania

References

[1] Clerico A, Giannoni A, Vittorini S, Passino C: Thirty years of the heart as an endocrine organ: physiological role and clinical utility of cardiac natriuretic hormones. Am J Physiol Heart Circ Physiol. 2011;301:H12–H20. doi:10.1152/ajpheart.00226.2011

[2] Cerillo AG, Storti S, Kallushi E, Haxhiademi D, Miceli A, Murzi M, Berti S, Glauber M, Clerico A, Iervasi G: The low triiodothyronine syndrome: a strong predictor of low cardiac output and death in patients undergoing coronary artery bypass grafting. Ann Thorac Surg. 2014;97:2089–2095. doi:10.1016/j.athoracsur.2014.01.049

[3] Del Ry S, Cabiati M, Clerico A: Recent advances on natriuretic peptide system: new promising therapeutic targets for the treatment of heart failure. Pharmacol Res. 2013;76:190–198. doi:10.1016/j.phrs.2013.08.006

[4] Canaris GJ, Manowitz NR, Mayor G, Ridgway EC: The Colorado thyroid disease prevalence study. Arch Intern Med. 2000;160:526–530. PMID: 10695693

[5] World Heart Federation Available from: http://www.world-heart-federation.org/cardiovascular-health/global-facts-map/. [Accessed: 26.08.2016]

[6] Rodondi N, Bauer DC, Cappola AR, Cornuz J, Robbins J, Fried LP, Ladenson PW, Vittinghoff E, Gottdiener JS, Newman AB: Subclinical thyroid dysfunction, cardiac function, and the risk of heart failure. The Cardiovascular Health Study. J Am Coll Cardiol. 2008;52:1152–1159. doi:10.1016/j.jacc.2008.07.009

[7] Nanchen D, Gussekloo J, Westendorp RG, Stott DJ, Jukema JW, Trompet S, Ford I, Welsh P, Sattar N, Macfarlane PW, Mooijaart SP, Rodondi N, de Craen AJ, PROSPER Group:

Subclinical thyroid dysfunction and the risk of heart failure in older persons at high cardiovascular risk. J Clin Endocrinol Metab. 2012;97:852–861. doi:10.1210/jc.2011-1978

[8] Galli E, Pingitore A, Iervasi G: The role of thyroid hormone in the pathophysiology of heart failure: clinical evidence. Heart Fail Rev. 2010;15:155–169. doi:10.1007/s10741-008-9126-6.

[9] Gerdes AM, Iervasi G. Thyroid replacement therapy and heart failure. Circulation. 2010;122:385–393. doi:10.1161/CIRCULATIONAHA.109.917922

[10] Fullerton MJ, Stuchbury S, Krozowski SZ, Funder JW. Altered thyroidal status and the in vivo synthesis of atrial natriuretic peptide in the rat heart. Mol Cell Endocrinol. 1990;69:227–233. PMID: 2139421

[11] Averyhart-Fullard V, Fraker LD, Murphy AM, Solaro RJ: Differential regulation of slow-skeletal and cardiac troponin I mRNA during development and by thyroid hormone in rat heart. J Mol Cell Cardiol. 1994;26:609–616. doi:10.1006/jmcc.1994.1073

[12] Tsai MJ, O'Malley BW: Molecular mechanisms of action of steroid/thyroid receptor superfamily members. Annu Rev Biochem. 1994;63:451–486. doi:10.1146/annurev.bi.63.070194.002315

[13] Davis PJ, Davis FB: Nongenomic actions of thyroid hormone. Thyroid. 1996;6:497–504. doi:10.1089/thy.1996.6.497

[14] Klein I, Ojamaa K: Thyroid hormone and the cardiovascular system. N Engl J Med. 2001;344:501–509. doi:10.1056/NEJM200102153440707

[15] Ribeiro RCJ, Apriletti JW, West BL, Wagner RL, Fletterick RJ, Schaufele F, Baxter JD: The molecular biology of thyroid hormone action. Ann N Y Acad Sci. 1995;758:366–389. PMID: 7625705

[16] Biondi B: Mechanisms in endocrinology: Heart failure and thyroid dysfunction. Eur J Endocrinol. 2012;167:609–618. doi:10.1530/EJE-12-0627

[17] Iervasi G, Pingitore A, Landi P, Raciti M, Ripoli A, Scarlattini M, L'Abbate A, Donato L: Low-T3 syndrome: a strong prognostic predictor of death in patients with heart disease. Circulation. 2003;107:708–713. doi:10.1161/01.CIR.0000048124.64204.3F

[18] Brenta G, Thierer J, Sutton M, Acosta A, Vainstein N, Brites F, Boero L, Gómez Rosso L, Anker S: Low plasma triiodothyronine levels in heart failure are associated with a reduced anabolic state and membrane damage. Eur J Endocrinol. 2011;164:937–942. doi:10.1530/EJE-11-0094.

[19] Pingitore A, Landi P, Taddei MC, Ripoli A, L'Abbate A, Iervasi G: Triiodothyronine levels for risk stratification of patients with chronic heart failure. Am J Med. 2005;118:132–136. doi:10.1016/j.amjmed.2004.07.052

[20] Nielsen CH, Brix TH, Leslie GQ: A role for autoantibodies in enhancement of pro-inflammatory cytokine responses to a self-antigen, thyroid peroxidase. Clin Immunol. 2009;133:218–227. doi:10.1016/j.clim.2009.07.014

[21] Wajner SM, Goemann IM, Bueno AL, Larsen PR, Maia AL: IL-6 promotes nonthyroidal illness syndrome by blocking thyroxine activation while promoting thyroid hormone inactivation in human cells. J Clin Invest. 2011;121:1834–1845. doi:10.1172/JCI44678

[22] Stanciu AE, Serdarevic N, Hurduc AE, Stanciu MM: IL-4, IL-10 and high sensitivity-CRP as potential serum biomarkers of persistent/recurrent disease in papillary thyroid carcinoma with/without Hashimoto's thyroiditis. Scand J Clin Lab Invest. 2015;75:539–548. doi:10.3109/00365513.2015.1057895

[23] Lubrano V, Pingitore A, Carpi A, Iervasi G: Relationship between triiodothyronine and proinflammatory cytokines in chronic heart failure. Biomed Pharmacother. 2010;64:165–169. doi:10.1016/j.biopha.2009.09.001

[24] Ponikowski P, Voors AA, Anker SD, Bueno H, Cleland JG, Coats AJ, Falk V, González-Juanatey JR, Harjola VP, Jankowska EA, Jessup M, Linde C, Nihoyannopoulos P, Parissis JT, Pieske B, Riley JP, Rosano GM, Ruilope LM, Ruschitzka F, Rutten FH, van der Meer P: Authors/Task Force Members; Document Reviewers: 2016 ESC Guidelines for the diagnosis and treatment of acute and chronic heart failure: The Task Force for the diagnosis and treatment of acute and chronic heart failure of the European Society of Cardiology (ESC). Developed with the special contribution of the Heart Failure Association (HFA) of the ESC. Eur J Heart Fail. 2016;18:891–975. doi:10.1002/ejhf.592

[25] Luers C, Sutcliffe A, Binder L, Irle S, Pieske B: NT-proANP and NT-proBNP as prognostic markers in patients with acute decompensated heart failure of different etiologies. Clin Biochem. 2013;46:1013–1019. doi:10.1016/j.clinbiochem.2013.03.014

[26] Stanciu AE, Vatasescu RG, Stanciu MM, Iorgulescu C, Vasile AI, Dorobantu M: Cardiac resynchronization therapy in patients with chronic heart failure is associated with anti-inflammatory and anti-remodelling effects. Clin Biochem. 2013;46:230–234. doi: 10.1016/j.clinbiochem.2012.11.002.

[27] Christ-Crain M, Morgenthaler NG, Meier C, Muller C, Nussbaumer C, Bergmann A, Staub JJ, Muller B: Pro-A-type and N-terminal pro-B-type natriuretic peptides in different thyroid function states. Swiss Med Wkly. 2005;135:549–554. doi:2005/37/smw-11119

[28] Kato K, Murakami H, Isozaki O, Tsushima T, Takano K: Serum concentrations of ANP and BNP in patients with thyrotoxicosis. Endocr J. 2009;56:17–27. PMID: 18827406

[29] Pakula D, Marek B, Kajdaniuk D, Krysiak R, Kos-Kudla B, Pakula P, Gatnar A, Borgiel-Marek H, Nowak M, Sieminska L, Glogowska-Szeląg J, Ostrowska Z: Plasma levels of NT-pro-brain natriuretic peptide in patients with overt and subclinical hyperthyroidism and hypothyroidism. Endokrynol Pol. 2011;62:523–528. PMID: 22144219

[30] Stanciu AE, Hurduc AE, Stanciu MM: Effects of thyroid hormone withdrawal on natriuretic peptides during radioactive iodine therapy in female patients with differentiated thyroid cancer. Scand J Clin Lab Invest. 2016. doi: 10.1080/00365513.2016.1230883

[31] Brozaitiene J, Mickuviene N, Podlipskyte A, Burkauskas J, Bunevicius R: Relationship and prognostic importance of thyroid hormone and N-terminal pro-B-Type natriuretic peptide for patients after acute coronary syndromes: a longitudinal observational study. BMC Cardiovasc Disord. 2016;16:45. doi:10.1186/s12872-016-0226-2

[32] Biondi B, Bartalena L, Cooper DS, Hegedus L, Laurberg P, Kahaly GJ: The 2015 European Thyroid Association Guidelines on diagnosis and treatment of endogenous subclinical hyperthyroidism. Eur Thyroid J. 2015;4:149–163. doi:10.1159/000438750

[33] Danzi S, Klein I: Thyroid hormone and the cardiovascular system. Minerva Endocrinol. 2004;29:139–150. PMID: 15282446

[34] Biondi B, Kahaly GJ: Cardiovascular involvement in patients with different causes of hyperthyroidism. Nat Rev Endocrinol. 2010;6:431–443. doi:10.1038/nrendo.2010.105

[35] Biondi B, Palmieri EA, Fazio S, Cosco C, Nocera M, Sacca L, Filetti S, Lombardi G, Perticone F: Endogenous subclinical hyperthyroidism affects quality of life and cardiac morphology and function in young and middle-aged patients. J Clin Endocrinol Metab. 2000;85:4702–4705. doi:10.1210/jcem.85.12.7085

[36] Kirchhof P, Benussi S, Kotecha D, Ahlsson A, Atar D, Casadei B, Castella M, Diener HC, Heidbuchel H, Hendriks J, Hindricks G, Manolis AS, Oldgren J, Popescu BA, Schotten U, Van Putte B, Vardas P: Authors/Task Force Members; Document Reviewers. 2016 ESC Guidelines for the management of atrial fibrillation developed in collaboration with EACTS: The Task Force for the management of atrial fibrillation of the European Society of Cardiology (ESC) Developed with the special contribution of the European Heart Rhythm Association (EHRA) of the ESC Endorsed by the European Stroke Organisation (ESO). Europace. 2016;pii:euw295. doi:10.1093/europace/euw295

[37] Cini G, Carpi A, Mechanick J, Cini L, Camici M, Galetta F, Giardino R, Russo MA, Iervasi G: Thyroid hormones and the cardiovascular system: pathophysiology and interventions. Biomed Pharmacother 2009;63:742–753. doi:10.1016/j.biopha.2009.08.003

[38] Schultz M, Kistorp C, Raymond I, Dimsits J, Tuxen C, Hildebrandt P, Faber J: Cardiovascular events in thyroid disease: a population based, prospective study. Horm Metab Res 2011;43:653–659. doi:10.1055/s-0031-1283162

[39] Collet TH, Gussekloo J, Bauer DC, den Elzen WP, Cappola AR, Balmer P, Iervasi G, Asvold BO, Sgarbi JA, Volzke H, Gencer B, Maciel RM, Molinaro S, Bremner A, Luben RN, Maisonneuve P, Cornuz J, Newman AB, Khaw KT, Westendorp RG, Franklyn JA, Vittinghoff E, Walsh JP, Rodondi N: Thyroid Studies Collaboration: Subclinical hyperthyroidism and the risk of coronary heart disease and mortality. Arch Intern Med 2012;172:799–809. doi:10.1001/archinternmed.2012.402

[40] Stanciu AE. Synthesis and applications of alpha/beta emitter-labelled nanoparticles. In: Llop J, Gomez-Vallejo V, editors. Isotopes in Nanoparticles: Fundamentals and Applications. Pan Stanford; 2016. pp. 383–427. doi:10.1201/b19950-16

[41] Siu CW, Yeung CY, Lau CP, Kung AW, Tse HF: Incidence, clinical characteristics and outcome of congestive heart failure as the initial presentation in patients with primary hyperthyroidism. Heart. 2007;93:483–487. doi:10.1136/hrt.2006.100628

[42] Biondi B, Klein I. Hypothyroidism as a risk factor for cardiovascular disease. Endocrine 2004;24:1–13. doi:10.1385/ENDO:24:1:001

[43] Biondi B, Palmieri EA, Lombardi G, Fazio S: Subclinical hypothyroidism and cardiac function. Thyroid. 2002;12:505–510. doi:10.1089/105072502760143890

[44] Biondi B: Cardiovascular effects of mild hypothyroidism. Thyroid. 2007;17:625–630. doi:10.1089/thy.2007.0158

[45] Klein I, Danzi S: Thyroid disease and the heart. Circulation. 2007;116:1725–1735. doi: 10.1161/CIRCULATIONAHA.106.678326

[46] Chaker L, Baumgartner C, den Elzen WP, Ikram MA, Blum MR, Collet TH, Bakker SJ, Dehghan A, Drechsler C, Luben RN, Hofman A, Portegies ML, Medici M, Iervasi G, Stott DJ, Ford I, Bremner A, Wanner C, Ferrucci L, Newman AB, Dullaart RP, Sgarbi JA, Ceresini G, Maciel RM, Westendorp RG, Jukema JW, Imaizumi M, Franklyn JA, Bauer DC, Walsh JP, Razvi S, Khaw KT, Cappola AR, Völzke H, Franco OH, Gussekloo J, Rodondi N, Peeters RP: Thyroid studies collaboration: Subclinical hypothyroidism and the risk of stroke events and fatal stroke: An individual participant data analysis. J Clin Endocrinol Metab. 2015;100:2181–2191. doi:10.1210/jc.2015-1438

[47] Brenta G, Mutti LA, Schnitman M, Fretes O, Perrone A, Matute ML: Assessment of left ventricular diastolic function by radionuclide ventriculography at rest and exercise in subclinical hypothyroidism, and its response to L-thyroxine therapy. Am J Cardiol. 2003;91:1327–1330. PMID: 12767425

[48] Ripoli A, Pingitore A, Favilli B, Bottoni A, Turchi S, Osman NF, De Marchi D, Lombardi M, L'Abbate A, Iervasi G: Does subclinical hypothyroidism affect cardiac pump performance? Evidence from a magnetic resonance imaging study. J Am Coll Cardiol. 2005;45:439–445. doi:10.1016/j.jacc.2004.10.044

[49] Ning N, Gao D, Triggiani V, Iacoviello M, Mitchell JE, Ma R, Zhang Y, Kou H: Prognostic role of hypothyroidism in heart failure: a meta-analysis. Medicine (Baltimore). 2015;94:e1159. doi:10.1097/MD.0000000000001159

[50] Biondi B, Cooper DS: The clinical significance of subclinical thyroid dysfunction. Endocr Rev. 2008;29:76–131. doi:10.1210/er.2006-0043

[51] Tiryakioglu SK, Tiryakioglu O, Ari H, Basel MC, Ozkan H, Bozat T: Left ventricular longitudinal myocardial function in overt hypothyroidism: a tissue Doppler echocar-

diographic study. Echocardiography. 2010;27:505–511. doi:10.1111/j.1540-8175.2009.01043.x

[52] Cooper DS, Biondi B: Subclinical thyroid disease. Lancet. 2012;379:1142–1154. doi: 10.1016/S0140-6736(11)60276-6

[53] Ravzi S, Ingoe L, Keeka G, Oates C, McMillan C, Weaver JU: The beneficial effect of L-thyroxine on cardiovascular risk factors, endothelial function and quality of life in subclinical hypothyroidism: randomized, crossover trial. J Clin Endocrinol Metab. 2007;92:1715–1723. doi:10.1210/jc.2006-1869

[54] Pearce SH, Brabant G, Duntas LH, Monzani F, Peeters RP, Razvi S, Wemeau JL. 2013 ETA Guideline: Management of Subclinical Hypothyroidism. Eur Thyroid J. 2013;2:215–228. doi:10.1159/000356507

[55] Gerdes A: Restoration of thyroid hormone balance: a game changer in the treatment of heart failure? Am J Physiol Heart Circ Physiol. 2015;308:H1–10. doi:10.1152/ajpheart.00704.2014

[56] Rajagopalan V, Gerdes AM: Role of thyroid hormones in ventricular remodeling. Curr Heart Fail Rep. 2015;12:141–149. doi:10.1007/s11897-014-0246-0

[57] Cokkinos DV, Chryssanthopoulos S: Thyroid hormones and cardiac remodeling. Heart Fail Rev. 2016;21:365–372. doi:10.1007/s10741-016-9554-7

[58] Martinez F: Thyroid hormones and heart failure. Heart Fail Rev. 2016;21:361–364. doi: 10.1007/s10741-016-9556-5

[59] Pingitore A, Nicolini G, Kusmic C, Iervasi G, Grigolini P, Forini F: Cardioprotection and thyroid hormones. Heart Fail Rev. 2016; 21:391–399. doi:10.1007/s10741-016-9545-8